O A P ⌣ L
OXFORD AMERICAN PALLIATIVE CARE LIBRARY

Grief and Bereavement in the Adult Palliative Care Setting

O A P C L
OXFORD AMERICAN PALLIATIVE CARE LIBRARY

Grief and Bereavement in the Adult Palliative Care Setting

E. Alessandra Strada, PhD, FT, MSCP

Adjunct Professor
The California Institute of Integral Studies
Faculty, Post-doctoral Psychopharmacology
Alliant University
San Francisco, California

Executive Series Editor
Russell K. Portenoy, MD

Chairman of the Department of Pain Medicine & Palliative Care
Beth Israel Medical Center
New York, NY

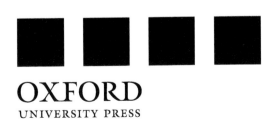

OXFORD
UNIVERSITY PRESS

OXFORD
UNIVERSITY PRESS

Oxford University Press is a department of the University of Oxford.
It furthers the University's objective of excellence in research, scholarship,
and education by publishing worldwide.

Oxford   New York
Auckland   Cape Town   Dar es Salaam   Hong Kong   Karachi
Kuala Lumpur   Madrid   Melbourne   Mexico City   Nairobi
New Delhi   Shanghai   Taipei   Toronto

With offices in
Argentina   Austria   Brazil   Chile   Czech Republic   France   Greece
Guatemala   Hungary   Italy   Japan   Poland   Portugal   Singapore
South Korea   Switzerland   Thailand   Turkey   Ukraine   Vietnam

Oxford is a registered trademark of Oxford University Press in the UK
and certain other countries.

Published in the United States of America by
Oxford University Press
198 Madison Avenue, New York, NY 10016

© Oxford University Press 2013

Library of Congress Cataloging-in-Publication Data
Strada, E. Alessandra.
Grief and bereavement in the adult palliative care setting / E. Alessandra Strada.
p. ; cm. — (Oxford American palliative care library)
Includes bibliographical references and index.
ISBN 978–0–19–976892–9 (alk. paper) — ISBN 978–0–19–990914–8 (alk. paper)
I. Title.   II. Series: Oxford American palliative care library.
[DNLM: 1. Bereavement.   2. Palliative Care—psychology.   3. Stress,
Psychological. BF 575.G7]
BF575.G7S764 2013
155.9'37—dc23
2013006037

9 8 7 6 5 4 3 2 1
Printed in the United States of America
on acid-free paper

Contents

Acknowledgments

I owe my greatest debt of gratitude to all the palliative care patients and their families with whom I have worked over the years. I have felt and continue to feel humbled and honored to be allowed into their intimate experience of grief and bereavement. It is to all of them that this book is dedicated.

I have been fortunate to have many wonderful mentors and colleagues who have been supportive, encouraging, and inspiring. I am especially grateful to Dr. Russell Portenoy, my former chairman, and all my former colleagues in the department of Pain Medicine and Palliative Care at Beth Israel Medical Center in New York. I have had the privilege to work with an extraordinary group of palliative care clinicians, whose commitment to this work has been a great source of inspiration. I would also like to thank my colleagues and friends at the California Institute of Integral Studies, in San Francisco and Alliant University, also in San Francisco. I am particularly grateful to all the students who have attended my class on the psychology of death and dying over the years, for participating with courage and authenticity in the exploration of their own experience of grief and bereavement.

I would like to thank everyone at Oxford for the continued support. I am most grateful to Andrea Seils, who has been a delight to work with.

My endless gratitude goes to my mother and my grandmother for their love and strength, and for teaching me the meaning of hope, resilience, and courage.

Most importantly, I thank my husband Tony. His love and support, his passion for life and wonderful sense of humor makes it all possible.

Definitions and Models

Chapter 1

Introduction

Focus Points

- Grief is the normal reaction to loss and it is characterized by physical, cognitive, psychological and spiritual manifestations.
- The impact of grief reactions on patients and families involves risk for significant distress and should never be underestimated.
- While grief has often been discussed in the context of the bereavement of surviving family members, the unique grief experience of palliative care patients requires specific focus, recognition, and support.
- Specialist-level palliative care clinicians should develop expertise in recognizing and supporting grief reactions and, when necessary, coordinating care with other providers.

The World Health Organization describes palliative care as "an approach that improves the quality of life of patients and their families facing the problems associated with life-threatening illness, through the prevention and relief of suffering by means of early identification and impeccable assessment and treatment of pain and other problems, physical, psychosocial, and spiritual."[1]

This definition recognizes that palliative care can be provided in conjunction with curative and life-prolonging treatment in order to improve quality of life and minimize side effects of treatment. Or it may become the main modality of care when patients are no longer receiving disease-modifying therapies and care becomes focused on improving quality of life, even as the illness progresses and patients continue to decline as they approach the end of life.[2]

While initially associated predominantly with cancer, palliative care is now increasingly being provided to patients with chronic, progressive pulmonary disorders, renal disease, heart failure, and nonmalignant neurological conditions.[3–6]

In 2004 leaders in palliative medicine from five major palliative care organizations within the United States developed a consensus document called The National Consensus Project for Quality Palliative Care. Eight core domains of palliative care were identified and defined along with clinical practice guidelines to provide quality care for patients and families by the members of the interdisciplinary palliative care team.

Grief and bereavement care are recognized as part of the psychological and psychiatric domain of palliative care, with the following recommendation: "Psychological and psychiatric issues are assessed and managed based upon the best available evidence, which is skillfully and systematically applied," *and*

"A grief and bereavement program is available to patients and families, based on the assessed need for service."[7]

Attention to grief reactions and bereavement is required for all specialist palliative care providers. The following guidelines for grief and bereavement care allow palliative care clinicians to meet best practice standards in this area (Table 1.1)

The initial fear of vulnerability that may occur after a diagnosis of a serious illness and the loss of the sense of well-being and safety is often the start of a long and challenging journey for patients and their caregivers. Therefore, grief reactions to these losses can be considered a common denominator for patients and caregivers during the different transitions of care from diagnosis, throughout treatment, to palliative and end-of-life care, and in bereavement, after the death of the patient.

The experience of loss is universal, but the experience and expression of grief is profoundly individual. Grief in advanced illness and in bereavement is a universal human experience, not an illness or a disease. And yet, clinicians' intuition and sensitivity may not be sufficient to meet the needs of patients and caregivers who are grieving the losses and implications of chronic and progressive illness. While the importance of empathy and compassion cannot be

---

Table 1.1 Grief and Bereavement Care Guideline and Criteria

- A grief and bereavement program is available to patients and families, based on the assessed need for service.

- The interdisciplinary team includes professionals with patient-population-appropriate education skills in the care of patients and families experiencing loss, grief, and bereavement.

- Bereavement services are recognized as a core component of the palliative care program.

- Bereavement services and follow-up are made available to the family for at least 12 months, or at least as is needed, after the death of the patient.

- Grief and bereavement risk assessment is routine, developmentally appropriate and ongoing for the patient and family throughout the illness trajectory, recognizing issues of loss and grief in living with a life-threatening illness.

- Clinical assessment is used to identify people at risk of complicated grief and bereavement, and its association with depression and co morbid complications.

- Information on loss and grief and the availability of bereavement support services, including those available through hospice and other community programs, is made routinely available to families before and after the death of the patient, as culturally appropriate and desired.

- Support and grief interventions are provided in accordance with developmental, cultural and spiritual needs, expectations and preferences of the family, including attention to the needs of siblings of pediatric patients and children of adult patients.

- Staff and volunteers who provide bereavement services receive ongoing education, supervision, and support.

- Referrals to health care professionals with specialized skills are made when clinically indicated.

Source: National Consensus Project for Quality Palliative Care. *Clinical Practice Guidelines for Quality Palliative Care.* Brooklyn, NY: National Consensus Project for Quality Palliative Care, 2004
Clinical Practice Guidelines for Quality Palliative Care, p. 25.

overestimated, the literature and clinical experience show that grief is a deceptively simple phenomenon. In reality, it is a multidimensional process with a course that is varied and complex. Grief reactions are shaped by personal and family history, psychological makeup, cultural norms and practices, and spiritual and religious beliefs and experiences.

Clinicians working in palliative care need specific education to understand and help manage grief in their patients and their caregivers. They need to recognize the impact of grief on coping skills, adjustment level, the decision-making process, and even treatment compliance. Furthermore, a significant body of research has shown, grief reactions may become pathological and warrant specific treatment.

Almost 2.5 million people die every year in the United States, leaving an overall even larger number of bereaved family members and other caregivers, friends, and colleagues having to cope with the death of someone close. Each year, approximately 800,000 people lose their spouse. Additionally, 10% of men and over 50% of women have lost their spouse at least once by age 65. Among the causes of death, heart disease was found to be the leading cause, followed by malignant neoplasm, cerebrovascular disease, and chronic respiratory disease.[8] These data suggest that most people who died spent at least some time in hospitals where they received treatment from medical and other health care providers. In many cases, grief becomes a regular element in the fabric of communications between patients, families, and the clinicians who care for them. Accordingly, it is important that clinicians develop adequate knowledge and understanding of the expression and manifestation of grief, as well as the ability to recognize when a pathological grieving process may be developing.[9]

The Palliative Care Setting

Palliative care can be provided in different inpatient and outpatient settings, including hospitals, clinics, nursing homes, or patients' home. The predominant model in the United States is the hospital-based palliative care consult team. Here, the primary treating team requests palliative care consultations for assistance addressing pain and other physical symptoms, as well as for social, psychological, and spiritual needs. Members of the palliative care team bring their expertise, ability, empathy, and compassion to the patient.

The sensitive and difficult conversations occurring between patients, caregivers, and providers regarding diagnosis and progression of illness, goals of care, or withdrawal of life-prolonging therapies may become catalysts for intense grief reactions, characterized by varying levels of emotional distress.[10] Clinicians who are able to recognize, validate, and support patients and families' experience and expression of grief will be more likely to establish a stronger connection with their patients and be a sustaining force during the ambiguous and challenging journey through illness.

Because the time available during the patient's hospitalization may be short, due to late referrals, discharge needs, and other system-related factors, clinicians need to provide grief screening, assessment, and intervention in a timely manner. Patients and caregivers may readily accept recommendations about pain and other symptoms, but they often need to develop a sense of trust before discussing their grief and emotional suffering. Thus, there is a need to integrate compassion, sensitivity, and the ability to quickly form trusting and empathic relationships in order to recognize, assess, and support grief reactions. Treatment plans can then be implemented to adequately minimize the impact of risk factors for severe grief reactions and to facilitate access to professional intervention, when needed.

Although the patient and family represent the unit of care, it is also crucial to recognize the patient's individual grief experience through the progression of illness. The palliative care patient's experience of grief needs to be understood, explored, and supported by members of the team. It needs to be differentiated from that of family members and other caregivers because it has unique features that often need to be approached differently. Accordingly, clinicians face the challenge to facilitate and support expression of grief in the family system, while ensuring that individual needs of patients and individual needs of each family member are recognized and addressed.

Effects of Grief

While grief is a natural response to loss, it has the potential to cause significant impairment and disability. Research has shown grief in bereavement can be associated with severe emotional distress, an increased risk for major depressive episodes, severe gastrointestinal symptoms, insomnia, anxiety, and even temporary perceptual disturbances, such as visual and auditory hallucinations.[19] Research has also shown that bereaved survivors have higher mortality rates from cardiovascular disease and infectious diseases than control participants.[20] Loss of a spouse is associated with increased mortality in surviving spouses,[21–24] and in widowers it has been associated with a 40% increase in mortality rates compared to controls.[25] Among bereaved men, harmful alcohol use and dependence symptoms are higher and may represent a mediator factor in increased mortality rates.[26] Suicide can be an extreme consequence of bereavement for some individuals.[27] In particular, bereaved elderly tend to be at greater risk for suicide given higher rates of social isolation and depression, especially if they have cared for a family member during a long illness.[28,29] Psychiatric illness, especially major depression and posttraumatic stress disorder, is one of the most common consequences of bereavement.[30,31] Complicated grief, a pathological form of grief reaction, has been associated with increased risk for major depressive disorder, posttraumatic stress disorder, generalized anxiety disorder, panic disorder, hypertension, cardiac events, and overall significantly reduced quality of life.[32–34]

While bereaved caregivers have been most studied, patients who are grieving their loss of health or their approaching death may experience intense preparatory grief and distress. Distressing effects of grief often overlap with other psychiatric disorders, making diagnosis challenging. As a result, grief reactions are often unrecognized and may even remain undiagnosed when they reach clinical significance. For example, it is important to recognize whether a patient with advanced illness is experiencing intense grief or depression.

Similarly, it is important that palliative care team members are able to identify family members at risk for complicated grief and bereavement-related major depression. Preexisting risk factors, including psychiatric vulnerability, psychosocial stressors, lack of financial resources, and lack of social support need to be considered in every evaluation, due to their potential to increase distress in grievers.

Definitions

Following is a brief description of grief reactions and grief-related terms commonly utilized in the literature and in clinical settings (Table 1.2).

Normal or Uncomplicated Grief

Grief is generally defined as the normal reaction to a loss that has significant emotional impact. The losses experienced by patients and caregivers in the palliative care setting are progressive and increasingly challenging, with the potential to elicit profound grief reactions. In this book, normal grief is used to indicate the expected cluster of physical, emotional, cognitive, spiritual, and interpersonal reactions experienced by patients with advanced illness and their caregivers.[12] The duration and intensity of the distress is a function of many variables that will be discussed, but it is important to emphasize that a certain

Table 1.2 Definitions	
Grief	Normal reaction to any significant loss. Physical, cognitive, psychological, and spiritual manifestations experienced as a reaction to loss.
Bereavement	The state of having experienced the death of someone close.
Mourning	The internal process of grieving to adapt to the death. It also refers to the outward manifestation of grief.
Anticipatory or preparatory grief	The grief experienced by family members before the death of a loved one from advanced illness The grieving process experienced by patients with advanced illness before they die.
Complicated grief or prolonged grief disorder	A multitude of severely distressing symptoms, including psychiatric presentations that indicate that the griever is "stuck" and the mourning process is not moving along. Complicated grief requires professional evaluation and intervention.
Disenfranchised grief	Losses are not supported or sanctioned by society (death of a married lover), that are not typically recognized as losses (death of a pet, spontaneous miscarriages), or losses that carry significant stigma (loss of a loved one by suicide, or lethal injection for a prisoner).
Chronic sorrow	Intense, prolonged sadness from losses caused by long, progressive, and debilitating illness. Can be experienced by both patients and caregivers.

level of distress is to be expected, or should at least be considered completely normal.

Bereavement

The term *bereavement* refers to the state of having experienced the loss to death of someone close.[13] Grief-focused care for caregivers should begin at the first contact with the palliative care team. It involves assessment of risk factors that may complicate bereavement. In addition, providing ongoing support to caregivers who are particularly at risk before and after the patient's death may be especially valuable.

Mourning

The term *mourning* is often used in the context of bereavement to indicate the process of integrating grief from the loss.[14,15] In essence, while bereavement indicates the state of having lost someone close, mourning refers to the emotional processing of the grief from that loss. It is also used to refer to the practical processing of that grief, such as funerals and memorial services.

Anticipatory or Preparatory Grief

These terms are often used interchangeably, both referring to the grieving process that occurs prior to the actual death[15] and is experienced by both patients and caregivers. More recently, the term *preparatory grief* has been used to specifically indicate the normal and expected grieving process experienced by patients with advanced illness as they are adjusting to the reality of advanced illness and their own death (see Chapter 6).

Complicated Grief or Prolonged Grief Disorder

Both terms, developed by two separate research groups (see Chapter 4), refer to the development of grief into a progressive pathological process. They indicate the prolonged and severe morbidity caused by grief that is not effectively processed and integrated by an individual after the death of someone close. As a result, the griever is symbolically "stuck" in the grieving process and continues to experience distressing symptoms that cause severe and disabling impairment long after the loss has occurred.[16] There is emerging evidence that complicated grief can also be experienced by patients with medical and advanced illness (see Chapter 4).

Chronic Sorrow

The term *chronic sorrow* was initially used to describe normal grief reactions in parents with children affected by severe developmental disability.[17] It is also used to indicate the ongoing and profound sadness caused by losses that are progressive or ambiguous in nature, as in patients with chronic, progressive disease, such as Parkinson's disease, amyotrophic lateral sclerosis, or dementia. In essence, chronic sorrow is intended to describe ongoing grief due to an ongoing living loss. As such, chronic sorrow can be experienced by both patients and caregivers, and it can contribute to the development of compassion fatigue in family caregivers. People experiencing chronic sorrow often describe the contrast between their life and what they expect life should have or could have been as the core of their emotional pain.

Disenfranchised Grief

Originated by Doka,[18] grief is disenfranchised when it occurs for losses that are not supported or recognized by societal norms. Therefore, the griever has less social permission to express grief. Grieving a miscarriage, the loss of a pet, or the death of a loved one in prison are examples of disenfranchised grief. The progressive and ambiguous losses caused by Alzheimer's disease and other types of dementia often create disenfranchised grief in caregivers. Clinicians should be able to recognize the disruptive nature of a grieving process that is forced into hiding. In the palliative care setting, those at risk for disenfranchised grief may be patients' ex-spouses, or spouses from a second marriage who have a strained relationship with the patients' children. Or it could be an estranged relative who is now seeking to reconnect with the patient and is not welcome by other family members. Disenfranchised grievers may describe feeling "not wanted" by other family members and therefore feel the necessity to grieve alone. Clinicians may also be at risk for disenfranchised grief, if they work in an environment where the emotional impact of their patients' death is minimized or ignored.

Nature and Meaning of Loss: Physical, Symbolic, and Ambiguous Losses

To understand grief, it is important to understand the nature of loss and review the main types of losses commonly experienced by patients and caregivers in the palliative care setting. A loss capable of causing a grief reaction can be understood as the experience of being deprived of something important.[11] Losses are commonly divided into two general categories: physical losses and symbolic losses. Some authors also refer to symbolic losses as psychosocial losses.

Physical losses involve the loss of something tangible. Losing limbs in an accident or losing a loved one to death are dramatic examples of physical losses.[12,13] Losing a breast due to breast cancer surgery is also a physical loss. Symbolic losses involve the loss of something that is mainly psychosocial in nature. Getting a divorce, losing a job, losing a friendship, or retiring are examples of symbolic losses.[14,15] Being diagnosed with a chronic pain syndrome, a life-limiting illness, transitioning from a curative to a palliative care modality, or transitioning to hospice care can also represent symbolic losses. What is lost is the hope that treatment will cure the illness and that life will just go back to the way things were before the illness diagnosis. While symbolic losses may not be as obvious as physical losses, they may cause severe emotional pain. For a patient with breast cancer, while losing a breast represents a physical loss, the symbolic loss of what the breast represents often generates even greater grief. In palliative care patients, symbolic losses are often superimposed on the ongoing physical losses resulting from worsening illness.

The implications or consequences of a loss, either physical or symbolic, is considered a *secondary loss*. This is illustrated by the example of a 45-year-old patient diagnosed with advanced colon cancer. He is a married man with school-age children and is the main provider in the family. After receiving the diagnosis he may grieve the loss of health and loss of the hope that life will continue without "bad news." The diagnosis represents a symbolic loss. However, he may also grieve the consequences, or secondary losses, associated with the diagnosis. For example, an inability to continue working full time because of illness or treatment side effects may cause loss of income, with negative effects for the family. The patient may also experience loss of status and role in the family as the main provider. As a result, his struggle to integrate the new reality of being a patient with cancer is compounded by the challenge to his preexisting sense of personal identity and the compounding effects of secondary losses. Providing adequate support to this patient requires an understanding of these effects together with a thorough exploration of all the layers of grief present and developing.

Some patients develop a very pragmatic and matter-of-fact approach to the actual diagnosis of serious illness and may be described as coping well, in control, and so on. However, the experience of grief may primarily relate to the consequences of the diagnosis and the practical and symbolic ways it affects their life. Such is the case of an 82-year-old patient recently diagnosed with metastatic ovarian cancer who was admitted to the hospital due to uncontrolled pain and overall physical decline.

This patient lived alone and valued her independence above all. Her oncologist told her she was too debilitated to tolerate disease-modifying treatment, and the focus of care should be on relieving pain and other symptoms. Upon hearing about her diagnosis and poor prognosis, the patient immediately asked whether she could be discharged home. She commented that she was not shocked to hear about her diagnosis because she had lived a long life and expected "something would happen at some point." She further commented that she was terrified by the thought that she would not be able to go back home and live independently. She stated, "I have always been the strong, independent type. I have always lived alone. If I cannot be that person, who am I going to be?" In working with this patient, it became clear that while she was relatively able to process losses related to the diagnosis of advanced cancer and her approaching death she was grieving the loss of her sense of identity and control. Her most severe grief was caused by a series of symbolic losses and the implications of such losses, i.e. losing the ability to continue living alone profoundly threatened her sense of self. Therefore, rather than making assumptions, clinicians should explore the meaning of the illness for each patient and family and understand how they experience and express grief.

The concept of *ambiguous loss*, originated and developed by Pauline Boss[16–18] is relevant to the palliative care setting. It refers to losses where grievers cannot develop a full sense of closure, due to the particular circumstances of the loss. For example, if a family member goes missing in a war zone and the body is never found, or a child is kidnapped and never found, it may never be possible to face the reality of the death because of the lack of a physical body. Accordingly, an inability to proceed with the processing of grief may occur.

In the palliative care setting, common ambiguous losses are those where the loved one is physically present but psychologically absent. For example, patients with Alzheimer's disease are physically present but progressively lose the ability to interact and connect with their loved ones. As a result, the caregiver begins the grieving process for the loss of the "person" before the actual death occurs. Similarly, caregivers of patients in a persistent vegetative state face the challenge of grieving the end of the relationship with the patient *as they knew it*, while seeing and caring for the physical body. The daughter of a patient with advanced dementia described her struggle in the following terms: "I already lost my mother, one piece at a time. But I see her body every day. And every day, when I first see her, I have a moment of confusion, and then hope. Hope that she will finally recognize me and we will all wake up from this nightmare. Here, the nurses are nice and they tell me she is peaceful. That I should be happy she has no pain and she is peaceful. I don't think people understand that this is constant torture. Is my mother dead? Is she alive? I don't know. I can't move on, because she is still here. But she is not. Her face is beautiful, no wrinkles. She looks like she could wake up any time. This is the worst type of torture. I am still mad at her for the past, but it is too late. I cannot bury her; I cannot bring her back. We are all stuck in this limbo, like emotional zombies" (verbatim, transcribed from a recorded therapy session).

Grieving may also be complicated by aspects of the relationship between patients and caregivers. Often, the person who has died is referred to as "the loved one," implying that the grief reactions in bereavement are the result of losing someone who is loved. However, in the palliative care setting, clinicians see a "snapshot in time" of a long and complex story of family dynamics and relationships. Often, the relationship between patients and caregivers has been complicated by a history of emotional or physical abuse, addiction, chronic mental illness, or overall maladaptive and unsupportive communication. As a result, the predominant emotion in some relationships may be resentment, and not necessarily love. In essence, the "loved one" is often "not just" the loved one. Still, family members may care for patients out of a sense of responsibility, guilt, or hope for reconciliation. Love may certainly be part of the picture, but it may be clouded by strong contrasting emotions (see also discussion on ambivalence in Chapter 2). In these circumstances, patients and caregivers may be more vulnerable to suffering and in need of support.[35]

Grief reactions in palliative care patients and their caregivers are complex and they have the potential to create distress in ways that are often not immediately obvious. Thus, it is essential that palliative care clinicians do not develop preconceived ideas about the nature and development of grief. Instead, there needs to be an in-depth curiosity, analysis, and understanding of the aspects and layers of grief reactions. This will allow implementation of a plan of support and treatment that is meaningful and clinically sound.

References

1. Sepulveda C, Marlin A, Yoshida T. Palliative care: The World Health Organization's global perspective. *J Pain Symptom Manage* 2002;24(2):91–6.

2. Morrison RS, Meier DE. Clinical practice: palliative care. *N Engl J Med* 2004;350(25):2582–90.

3. Hardin KA, Meyers F, Louie S. Integrating palliative care in severe chronic obstructive lung disease. *COPD* 2008;5(4):207–20.

4. Cohen LM, Germain M, Poppel DM, et al. Dialysis discontinuation and palliative care. *Am J Kidney Dis* 2000;36:140–4.

5. Goodlin SJ, Hauptman PJ, Arnold R, et al. Consensus statement: palliative and supportive care in advanced heart failure. *J Cardiovasc Nurs* 2004;19:76–83.

6. Oliver D, Borasio GD, Walsh D, eds. *Palliative Care in Amyotrophic Lateral Sclerosis—From Diagnosis to Bereavement.* 2nd ed. Oxford, England: Oxford University Press; 2006.

7. National Consensus Project for Quality Palliative Care. *Clinical Practice Guidelines for Quality Palliative Care.* 2004 Brooklyn, NY: National Consensus Project for Quality Palliative Care.

8. Heron M, Tejada-Vera B. Deaths: leading causes for 2005. National Vital Statistics Reports Vol. 58, # 8. Available at: http://198.246.98.21/nchs/data/nvsr/nvsr58/nvsr58_08.pdf. Accessed September 25, 2010.

9. Moon PJ. Untaming grief? For palliative care physicians. *Am J Hosp Palliat Care* 2011;28(8):569–72.

10. Hudson PL, Thomas K, Trauer T, Remedios C, Clarke D. Psychological and social profile of family caregivers on commencement of palliative care. *J Pain Symptom Manage* 2011;41(3):522–34.

11. Clieren M. *Bereavement and Adaptation: A Comparative Study of the Aftermath of Death.* Washington, DC: Hemisphere Publishing Corporation; 1993.

12. Stroebe M, Schut H, Stroebe W. Health outcomes of bereavement. *Lancet* 2007;370(9603):1960–73.

13. Raphael B, Dobson M. Bereavement. In: Harvey JH, Miller ED, eds. *Loss and Trauma.* Philadelphia, PA: Brunner Routledge Publishers; 2000:45–61.

14. Sprang G, McNeil J. *The Many Faces of Bereavement: The Nature and Treatment of Natural, Traumatic, and Stigmatized Grief.* New York: Brunner/Mazel Publishers; 1995.

15. Abi-Hashem N. Grief, loss, and bereavement: an overview. *J Psychol Christianity* 1999;18(4):309–29.

16. Attig T. *How We Grieve: Relearning the World.* New York: Oxford University Press; 1996.

17. Boss P, Roos S, Harris DL. Grief in the midst of ambiguity and uncertainty. An exploration of ambiguous loss and chronic sorrow. In: Neimeyer RA, Harris DL, Winouker HR, Thornton GF, eds. *Grief and Bereavement in Contemporary Society: Bridging Research and Practice.* New York: Routledge; 2011:163–175.

18. Doka K. Disenfranchised grief: New directions, challenges, and strategies for practice. Champaign, IL: Research Press. 2002.

19. Lindstrom TC. Immunity and health after bereavement in relation to coping. *Scand J Psychol* 1997;38:253–59.

20. Manor O, Eisenbach Z. Mortality after spousal loss: are there socio-demographic differences? *SocSci Med* 2003;56(2):405–13.

21. Hart CL, Hole DJ, Lawlor DA, et al. Effect of conjugal bereavement on mortality of the bereaved spouse in participants of the Renfrew/Paisley Study. *J Epidemiol Community Health* 2007;61(5):455–60.

22. Espinosa J, Evans WN. Heightened mortality after the death of a spouse: marriage protection or marriage selection? *J Health Econ* 2008;27(5):1326–42.

23. Helsing KL, Szklo M. Mortality after bereavement. *Am J Epidemiol* 1981;114:41–52.

24. Rando T. *Treatment of Complicated Mourning.* Champaign, IL: Research Press Company; 1993.

25. Prigerson HG, Frank E, Kasl S, et al. Complicated grief and bereavement-related depression as distinct disorders: preliminary empirical validation in elderly bereaved spouses. *Am J Psychiatry* 1995;152:22–30.

26. Pilling J, Konkoly TB, Demetrovics Z, Kopp MS. Alcohol use in the first three years of bereavement: a national representative survey. *Subst Abuse Treat Prev Policy* 2012;7(1):3

27. Jones DR, Goldblatt PO. Causes of death in widowers and spouses. *J Biosocial Science* 1987;19:107–21.

28. Ajdacic-Gross V, Ring M, Gadola E, et al. Suicide after bereavement: an overlooked problem. *Psychol Med* 2008;38(5):673–6.

29. Erlangsen A, Jeune B, Bille-Brahe U, et al. Loss of partner and suicide risks among oldest old: a population-based register study. *Age Ageing* 2004;33(4):378–83.

30. Zhang B, Mitchell SL, Bambauer KZ, et al. Depressive symptoms trajectories and associated risks among bereaved Alzheimer disease caregivers. *Am J Geriatr Psychiatry* 2008;16(2):145–55.

31. Macias C, Jones J, Harvey P, et al. Bereavement in the context of serious mental illness. *Psychiatr Serv* 2004;55(4):421–6.

32. Nolen-Hoeksema S, Larson J. *Coping with Loss.* London: *Lawrence Erlbaum Associates*; 1999.

33. Murphy SA, Johnson LC, Chung IJ, et al. The prevalence of PTSD following the violent death of a child and predictors of change 5 years later. *J Trauma Stress* 2003;16(1):17–25.

34. Ott, CH. The impact of complicated grief on mental and physical health at various points in the bereavement process. *Death Studies* 2003; 27(3): 249–272.

35. Strada EA. The helping professional's guide to end of life care. Oakland, CA: New Harbinger, 2013.

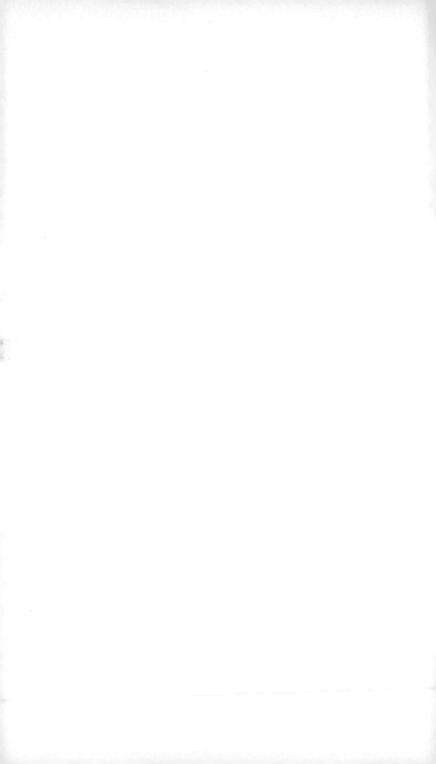

Chapter 2

Models of Grief and Relevance to the Palliative Care Setting

Focus Points

- Grief is a multifaceted process that does not follow stages or phases in a linear or predictable course.
- Some patients and caregivers experience profound and prolonged distress during normal grief and mourning; others appear to be adjusting relatively quickly and without significant distress.
- Contrary to early beliefs, overt expression of intense affect and distress during grief reactions is not a necessary requirement for effective integration of loss and adjustment.
- While early models emphasized the need to disconnect emotionally from the deceased, current conceptualizations recognize the importance of maintaining and evolving supportive emotional ties with the person who died.

Early developers of grief models differed in their conceptualization of how grief can be processed, but they generally agreed on the existence of stages or phases of grief that individuals experience during the mourning process. Mourning, the psychological process of adapting to loss of a loved one to death, was considered to be characterized by "grief work," an intense period of emotional pain necessary for "working through" the pain of grief and thought to be essential for the normal functioning of the psyche. It was also believed that absence of expressed grief in bereavement was not a typical response and was due to either lack of strong attachment to the deceased or to protective suppression of grief.[1] As such, absence of grief was believed to be counterproductive and potentially damaging.

The growing body of bereavement research has not supported the existence of sequential stages or phases of grief. Therefore, recent conceptualizations emphasize the uniqueness of the grieving process for each patient and each caregiver, and the importance of understanding the nature of the multiple variables that affect the grieving process. Individuals develop personal grieving styles that are strongly influenced by cultural and psychospiritual factors and may or may not include overt expression of strong negative affect. More recently, patients' preparatory grief has become the focus of empirical research, allowing for an expanded understanding of existing frameworks.

Mourning, Melancholia, and Ambivalence

Freud described the potential disruptive impact of bereavement-related grief. His observation of the different ways his patients reacted to and adjusted to the loss of someone close prompted his differentiation between mourning, as an adaptive process, and melancholia, identified as a pathological manifestation of grief.[2,3] Mourning is described as a long and very demanding process, involving a significant amount of time and emotional energy.

According to his model, an adaptive reaction to grief involves a progressive and continuous detachment from the memories and emotions connected to the loved one who died. Thus, the bereaved individual is supposed to disinvest emotional energy attached to the deceased and reinvest it into other people. Freud was advocating for emotional detachment from the deceased; however, he also postulated that metaphorically, nonpathological mourning allows the survivor to progressively internalize aspects of the deceased. This internalization allows the bereaved survivor not only to survive the pain of loss but also to feel secure enough to invest emotional energy into other people. Freud stated this theory in *Totem and Taboo*: "Mourning has quite a precise task to perform; its function is to detach the survivors' memories and hopes from the dead" (1912, p. 65). Current understanding of grief and bereavement have emphasized that mourners do not necessarily need to detach from the memories of the deceased, as much as integrate the relationship into a new framework that is nurturing and supportive.[4] The ability to maintain such supportive connection with the memory and legacy of the deceased in an important aspect of many people's bereavement.

Freud also differentiated mourning from melancholia, his term for depression, as occurring when the process of mourning fails. He attributed melancholia to a number of intrapsychic elements, especially preexisting ambivalence in the relationship.

Considering ambivalence in the relationship prior to the death as a risk factor that may complicate the grieving process has much contemporary clinical relevance in the palliative care setting, both for patients and caregivers. Ambivalence involves feeling not only positive emotions toward someone who is dying but also significant negative feelings that are not easy to process and perhaps have never been acknowledged or explored. This scenario is not uncommon in the palliative care setting. Consider the following case example.

Rose is the primary caregiver for her husband, who has advanced prostate cancer. The couple have been married for more than 20 years and have three children. Rose appears very dedicated to her husband's care and spends most of the time at the hospital, in his room, but mostly reading and talking on the phone to her friends. The palliative care team notices that Rose has positioned her chair as far from the bed as possible and nursing staff report that she rarely approaches the bed. When she does go close to help her husband eat his meals, it appears she tries very carefully not to touch him. When the patient is interviewed alone, he comments that his wife is a cold and detached woman, who is not able to provide comfort to him. In an attempt to obtain a clearer picture of the family dynamic, the wife is interviewed alone. She reveals that her husband is an alcoholic who has been sober for the past 5 years. However, she shares with the team that during the years when he was drinking, he was verbally and physically abusive toward her and the children. She explains that he hit her while she was pregnant and as a result she miscarried.

Rose states clearly that she has never completely forgiven her husband for the abuse. In tears, she says that watching her husband lying in bed, vulnerable, powerless, and needy, she feels torn by many contrasting emotions. She concludes saying that she loves him for the person he has become, but she hates him for the hurt he caused her. She adds that she is worried about managing her emotions after his death, because she feels that after he dies she will be forever alone with her feelings and there will be no resolution.

Ambivalence is clearly present in the relationship between Rose and her dying husband. Her expressed concern about processing her complex emotions after his death indicates that ambivalence is a significant risk factor with the potential to negatively affect her bereavement. Clinicians should recognize this risk factor, and psychological support should be provided to Rose during caregiving and into bereavement. Rose started psychotherapy with a member of the palliative care team and continued after her husband's death. Providing psychological care to Rose prior to the actual death was essential. It allowed her to process some of her feelings of resentment and guilt that were preventing her from connecting emotionally with her husband. Since her stated goal was to achieve some peace around the past and be able to express her love to him before his death, the therapy focused on achieving this goal.

Absent Grief

Along with the Freudian idea that recovering from bereavement involves long and painful work, in the late 19th century Helene Deutsch proposed that grief must be openly expressed and described the absence of such expression as a potentially pathological response.[1] She described mourning as a process that needs to be brought to completion and "accomplished," because "unmanifested grief will be found expressed to the full in some way or other" (p. 13).

Modern approaches to grief and bereavement have indicated the necessity to deconstruct the concept of absent grief reactions. Overt expression of emotions traditionally associated with grief reactions, such as crying and inability to continue to function, are primarily a function of individual grieving styles (see Chapter 3). Lack of expression of strong negative affect does not necessarily imply that mourning is not taking place. Once again, accurate screening and individualized assessment can help the clinician understand whether the individual's reactions are maladaptive or simply a manifestation of a personal and non-pathological style.

The Distress Caused by Normal Grief

The first psychiatric study of normal, non-pathological grief reactions was published by Erich Lindemann in 1944, after a fire that caused the death of nearly 500 people at the Coconut Grove, a night club in Boston.[5] His paper "The Symptomatology and Management of Acute Grief" described the reactions of bereaved family members. While the study contained methodological limitations, Lindemann described clusters of symptoms that can be observed in people during the acute phase of grief and are considered normal aspects of grief:

- Distressing physical symptoms that include an initial sense of numbness
- Preoccupation with sad memories about the deceased
- Guilt
- Anger toward others
- Loss of regular patterns of conduct

Lindemann originated the term "grief work," which appropriately describes the processing of grief as "work," involving the intense mobilization of emotional, cognitive, physical, and spiritual energy to process and integrate the loss.

When educating patients and caregivers about grief, it may be helpful to use the expression "grief work" to explain and normalize the variety of distressing physical and emotional symptoms that may characterize the grieving process. Patients and family members experiencing high levels of distress usually feel reassured knowing there is a valid explanation for how difficult grieving feels. To some people, it literally feels like "work" and, as such, it is a burden that influences many daily activities.

However, not all grievers will relate to the concept that grief is hard work. For some bereaved individuals, adaptation and coping do not necessarily imply a very long and excruciatingly painful review of memories attached to the deceased. They seem able to continue functioning in their environment and report feeling "ok" relatively soon after the loss. It is important that such individuals do not feel that they are "doing something wrong" or that they are not grieving appropriately.

As noted previously, early grief theories identified the ability to emotionally detach or let go of the deceased as an essential task for effective mourning. According to Lindemann's model, grief work involved three main tasks: "emancipation from the deceased, readjustment to a world without the deceased, and formation of new relationships." The concept of emancipation from the deceased needs to be understood in the context of the early psychoanalytic theory. Current understanding of grief and bereavement has actually highlighted that grievers do not so much withdraw emotional energy as modify the sense of their relationship with the deceased. The goal is not to "forget" the person who died but to have progressively more emotional energy available to invest in other activities and relationships.

The Dimensions of Denial

In 1961, George Engel, one of the most important figures in psychosomatic medicine and developer of the biopsychosocial model, wrote a classic paper titled "Is Grief a Disease? A Challenge for Medical Research."[6] In this work, Engel made several contributions to the study and understanding of the clinical manifestations of grief. He identified two major risk factors in the grieving process: inability to cry and identification with the deceased caused by guilt. Inability to cry refers to a situation when the griever feels like crying and that crying would be appropriate, but he or she is unable to do so. According to Engel, this situation may be caused by a high level of ambivalence in the relationship, which may not allow the griever to have access to a direct expression of emotions.

The second risk factor refers to a case in which the griever adopts some of the deceased's undesirable personality traits to symbolically strengthen the alliance and the bond with the deceased, even when the behavior is maladaptive.

Engel also contributed theories related to the concept of denial, differentiating denial of the death from denial of the loss or the emotions connected to the death. In the first case, a bereaved individual may deny that the death has occurred and continue to search for evidence that the loved one is still alive. In the second case, a bereaved individual may be able to cognitively understand and acknowledge that the death has occurred but may be unable to recognize and emotionally connect with emotions, significance, and overall impact of the death.

Attachment and Loss

The British psychoanalyst John Bowlby allowed for a further understanding of grief reactions through his conceptualization of attachment theory. According to Bowlby, humans have a natural propensity to form attachments to others. Based on his study of infants separated from their mothers and institutionalized, he described grief as a series of attachment behaviors performed after the loss of an object of attachment.[7,8] Bowlby described the mourning process as characterized by four phases:

1. Numbness and denial
2. Yearning and searching
3. Disorganization
4. Gradual reintegration

Bowlby also identified four patterns of early attachment that affect how people engage in relationships and that may determine the outcome of their mourning process.[9] Secure attachment usually translates into the ability to form intimate and trusting relationships. This attachment pattern does not mitigate the pain of grief if a loved one dies, but over time it can allow the bereaved to maintain a sense of psychological safety and integrity in the world and facilitate the adjustment process. Insecure attachment is dominated by a pattern of anxiety and inability to trust. Dependent attachment may result in dependent relationships with significant clinging behavior. Avoidant attachment may translate into relationship styles that value independence and self-sufficiency as a core value. A dependent attachment style, with high levels of dependency in the relationship, is now considered a possible risk factor for the development of complicated grief. Understanding the predominant attachment style of the patient and caregiver and related risk factors may allow clinicians to better direct grief and bereavement care.

Changes in the Assumptive World and Pathological Grief

Colin Parkes, a British psychiatrist who worked with Dame Cecily Saunders at St. Christopher's Hospice, described the bereaved individual's experience of loss as having the power to change the "assumptive world," meaning the set of beliefs, expectations, and thoughts about how the world functions or is supposed to function. The loss of a loved one shatters the set of familiar expectations and leaves the individual in an unfamiliar territory, where familiar assumptions are no longer valid.[10,11] During the mourning process, individuals face the task of symbolically creating a new view of the world, which may involve, in existential terms, developing a new way of "being in the world."

Parkes and Weiss[10] also identified three forms of pathological grief from unresolved bereavement:

- *Unexpected grief.* It results from a devastating, sudden, and traumatic loss that severely compromises the survivor's ability to use existing coping skills to adjust.
- *Conflicted grief.* It may develop in the context of a highly conflictual, ambivalent relationship with the deceased and may result in pining, severe anxiety, guilt, and yearning.
- *Chronic grief.* This pattern of pathological grief may develop from a relationship with the deceased characterized by high levels of emotional and practical dependency. Here, the bereaved feels unable to continue meeting the demands of everyday life without the emotional and concrete help of the deceased.

It is a recognized fact that serious and advanced illness has the power to "change the assumptive world" for patients, as well as their caregivers. Living with advanced illness involves the ability to manage a high level of ambiguity related to all aspects of care. As a result, patients and family members face the challenging task of constantly adapting to the evolving realities of the course of their illness, as well as their evolving sense of the world, of themselves, and of their future. And when the death of the patient occurs, the bereaved caregivers' assumptive world is often turned upside down, all over again.

The Dual-Process Model of Grief

While the process of recovering from a loss is highly individual and does not follow a predictable course, most bereaved individuals are eventually able to integrate the loss into their lives. Strobe and Shut[12-14] described this complex process as the "dual-process model of grief." The dual-process model of grief includes a loss-oriented response and a restoration-oriented response. While the former represents the active form of grieving and can be highly distressing, the latter runs parallel to it and involves the expression of active coping skills that allow the individual to process the loss and integrate it into his or her life. In clinical practice, grievers' expression of grief often alternate between periods focused on reviewing the loss and experiencing distress, and periods with a demonstrated ability to cope with the loss and integrate it is a meaningful way. This emotional and cognitive fluctuation from loss-oriented response to restoration-oriented response can often be observed in bereaved individuals but also in palliative care patients, as they attempt to process the implications of advanced illness: progression of disease, news that disease-modifying treatment is no longer an option, and possibility that death may be close. In this context, clinicians may observe that patients' responses do not always follow the same course and are likely to fluctuate. On some days they may appear completely immersed in the grieving process; other times their mood may be completely different and they may, for example, become focused on life-enhancing activities. As one patient with advanced cancer put it, "Sometimes I just need to take a break from feeling sad that I can't be cured and I am going to die. I have days when I just don't want to think about it. Those are the days I think about what I want to do now and I get busy thinking about changing the curtains in the living room. You just can't think about dying all the time." A bereaved woman whose partner died of lung cancer reflected, "I have days when I cannot do anything other than cry and miss her. I can go on like that for many days. And then I sometimes wake up and just don't feel as much pain and I think that I am going to make it and that it would be nice to visit some of the places we always wanted to go to and to learn to play a musical instrument."

Grief in Patients with Advanced Illness

Elisabeth Kubler-Ross was probably the first clinician to attempt a systematic study of grief reactions experienced by patients with terminal illness. On the basis of her interviews with patients who were approaching death, she developed the well-known stage model that describes patients' reactions as a linear sequence starting with denial, and followed by anger, bargaining, depression, and acceptance.[15] Her model, criticized for the sequential and fixed understanding of the stages, has not been supported by bereavement research or experience in clinical practice. However, the reactions she described can often be observed in patients with advanced illness and their caregivers, not as static stages, but as predominant behavioral patterns that may characterize the adaptation process.

The Study and Treatment of Complicated Mourning

Building on psychoanalytic and object relations theories, Therese Rando developed a comprehensive and clinically relevant model. Her model of mourning includes three phases: avoidance, confrontation, and accommodation.[16] Rando further identified six processes of mourning within the three phases[17] and described complications that may occur during each process and the therapeutic interventions that may minimize risk factors and morbidity for the griever. The concept of "process," rather than phase or stage, is more relevant to the realities of clinical practice because it emphasizes complexity, rather than linearity. These processes are as follows:

1. Recognize the loss
2. React to the separation
3. Recollect and re-experience the deceased and the relationship
4. Relinquish the old attachments to the deceased and the old assumptive world
5. Readjust to move adaptively into the new world without forgetting the old one
6. Reinvest

Rando also elaborated on a phenomenon that resonates with many grieving individuals, called subsequent temporary upsurges of grief (STUG). The term refers to the experience of acute, intense grief that may even occur several years after the loss of the loved one.[17] Anniversaries and other important dates or festivities are known for their potential to elicit profound sadness even several years after the death.[14] However, these intense reactions can be triggered and precipitated by several other factors, including seasons, memories, or music. Since they are not necessarily an indication of complicated grief, they should be considered normal in the absence of other factors that suggest a pathological process.

The Task Model: Grief Counseling and Grief Therapy

William Worden[18] described mourning as a process involving four main tasks:

1. Accepting the reality of the loss
2. Working through the pain of grief
3. Adjusting to a world without the deceased
4. Finding an enduring connection with the deceased in the midst of embarking on a new life

Worden emphasizes the tasks are not necessarily linear, nor are they to be understood as fixed stages, as some tasks can also occur concurrently.

Additionally, he differentiated between grief counseling, as a process of "helping people facilitate uncomplicated, or normal grief to a healthy adaptation to the task of mourning within a reasonable time frame," from grief therapy, which requires the "specialized techniques...that are used to help people with abnormal or complicated grief reactions" (p. 83). While Worden's model was developed to describe the grieving process after the loss of a loved one, it can be also meaningfully applied to patients with advanced illness and their process of adaptation to the difficult transitions of care common in the palliative care setting.[28]

The Meaning-Making Process in Mourning

In the last decade, Neimeyer and colleagues[19–21] have developed a model that emphasizes the importance of the process of making meaning of the loss, especially in circumstances of traumatic losses. The meaning-making process in the face of loss is individual and impacted by emotional, cognitive, cultural, and spiritual factors. The goal is for the mourner to integrate the loss into a personal narrative of one's life. This model is also relevant to the work with patients with advanced illness. The meaning-making process is, for many patients, an essential component of their processes of adaptation. During the journey from diagnosis to advanced illness and death, patients struggle to make meaning, or make sense of their experience, and integrate a new meaning into their lives, their sense of identity, and their personal narratives.

Continuing Bonds with the Deceased

This framework emphasizes the positive connection that continues to exist between many bereaved individuals and the deceased.[22] Unlike grief and bereavement models that describe the importance of withdrawing emotional energy from the deceased and reinvesting it in other objects of attachment, the continuing bond model recognizes that in many cases, the relationship with the loved one who died changes, but it does not end. It may become an internalized source of encouragement and enhance the life of the bereaved. This continued connection can be expressed in different ways, with some bereaved individuals writing letters to the deceased or engaging in imaginal conversations with the deceased. Clinicians must be able to recognize the difference between a positive transformation of the relationship as an adaptive response, and manifestations of complicated grief, where the bereaved is stuck in the grieving process. As a general indication, bereaved individuals who have been able to transform their relationship with the deceased in a positive way are progressively able to engage in life-enhancing activities and may feel stronger, supported, or protected by the loved one who died. On the contrary, bereaved individuals who are experiencing complicated grief display behaviors that may suggest attempts to continue the relationship with the deceased, but in fact they cause severe distress, such as distressing yearning, pining, and longing, with no experience of relief.[23]

Two-Track Model of Bereavement

According to this model, developed by Rubin in the early 1980s, effective management of bereavement requires not only attention to the biopsychosocial responses of the griever but should also explore the griever's relationship with the deceased, prior to the death and after the death. The uniqueness of the model lies in its recognition of the relationship with the deceased as an important element of interpersonal functioning affected by death, and constantly affecting the bereaved individual's ability to integrate the loss. As a result, clinical work to assist grievers will focus not only on exploring and supporting biopsychosocial function but also on exploring and addressing the relationship with the deceased prior to the death and its evolution after the death.[24,25] In both the biopsychosocial and relationship-with-the-deceased tracks, the clinician is encouraged to understand the extent of the griever's strengths and weaknesses and to facilitate processing traumatic experiences related to the death, promoting integration.

Resilience

Bonanno's empirical research on thousands of bereaved individuals has highlighted the role of resilience and adaptive suppression of emotions in the mourning process. Earlier conceptualizations of bereavement have not emphasized the role of personal resilience as a key factor in the mourning process, highlighting instead emotional and physical distress as necessary components of grief work. However, the majority of individuals interviewed in the course of Bonanno's research appeared to recover relatively quickly and to be able to return to prior levels of function without need for professional help and without overt expression of significant distress.[26,27] He identified three patterns of grief reactions: chronic grief, recovery, and resilience. People who experience chronic grief endure prolonged, debilitating distress for years and are often unable to return to their regular lives without professional help. The recovery pattern involves a more gradual course, with initial acute grief, followed by a progressive ability to continue on with life. Resilient grievers may experience pain from the loss, but they may not seem affected in a disabling way and may return to their lives relatively quickly.

Bonanno's framework helped expand the understanding of grief and bereavement as a multidimensional construct that may elicit unique sets of experience for different individuals. For some people, death of someone close will involve the experience of severe and prolonged distress; others may recover relatively quickly and with minimal distress involved. Personal variables, including the nature of the relationship with the deceased, will affect and determine the course of individual mourning. Describing a grieving family member or a patient as "resilient" has clearly positive connotations and acknowledges the person's ability to cope in the face of profound pain and loss. However, clinicians should be cautioned not to implicitly think that a so-called resilient style is "better" or somehow more desirable than a grieving style that involves more overt expression of distress. Once again, it is important to remember that there is no right way to grieve and that grief is a profoundly unique and personal experience that needs to be supported, and not pathologized, even when it involves profound distress. The challenge for clinicians is to identify the threshold beyond which grief becomes a disorder or triggers a disorder.

Clinicians in the palliative care setting will observe that grief reactions in patients and caregivers present with great variation. Familiarity with grief models and theories can provide a helpful theoretical framework for thinking about grief reactions. However, since there is no right or wrong way to grieve, clinicians must refrain from labeling or rating patients and families on the basis of their grief responses. Clinicians' initial goal should be to develop a full understanding of the human experience and expression of grief in its unique variations, refraining from making assumptions, assessing without judging, and offering support unconditionally.

References

1. Deutch H. Absence of grief. *Psychoanalytic Quarterly* 1937;6:12–22.

2. Freud S. Mourning and melancholia. In: Strachey J, trans-ed. *The Standard Edition of the Complete Psychological Works of Sigmund Freud*. Vol. 14. London: Hogarth; 1957:237–259.

3. Freud S. Totem and taboo. In: Strachey J, trans-ed. *The Standard Edition of the Complete Works of Sigmund Freud*. Vol. 13. London: Hogarth; 1955: 1–161.

4. Klass D, Silverman PR, Nickman SL, eds. *Continuing Bonds: New Understandings of Grief*. Philadelphia, PA: Taylor & Francis; 1996.

5. Lindemann E. The symptomatology and management of acute grief. *Am J Psychiatry* 1944;101:141–8.

6. Engel GL. Is grief a disease? A challenge for medical research. *Psychosomatic Med* 1961;23:18–22.

7. Bowlby J. Grief and mourning in infancy and early childhood. *Psychoanalytic Study Child* 1960;15:9–52.

8. Bowlby J. The making and breaking of affectional bonds: II. Some principles of psychotherapy. *Brit J Psychiatry* 1977;130:421–31.

9. Bowlby J. *Attachment and Loss: Vol. 3. Loss, Sadness, and Attachment*. New York: Basic Books; 1980.

10. Parkes CM, Weiss R. *Recovery from Bereavement*. New York: Basic Books; 1983.

11. Parkes CM. *Love and Loss: The Roots of Love and Its Complications*. New York: Rountledge; 2006.

12. Stroebe MS, Shut H. The dual process model of coping with bereavement: rational and description. *Death Studies* 1999;23:197–224.

13. Stroebe MS, Hansson RO, Stroebe W, Shut H, eds. *Handbook of Bereavement Research: Consequences, Coping, and Care*. Washington, DC: American Psychological Association; 2001.

14. Stroebe M, Schut H. The dual process model of coping with bereavement: a decade on. *Omega (Westport)* 2010;61(4):273–89.

15. Kubler-Ross E. *On Death and Dying.* New York: Touchstone; 1969.

16. Rando TA, ed. *Clinical Dimensions of Anticipatory Mourning.* Champaign, IL: Research Press; 2000.

17. Rando TA. *Treatment of Complicated Mourning.* Champaign, IL: Research Press; 1993.

18. Worden J. *Grief Counseling and Grief Therapy: A Handbook for the Mental Health Professional.* New York: Springer; 2009.

19. Neymeyer RA. Searching for the meaning of meaning: grief therapy and the process of reconstruction. *Death Studies* 2000;24(6):541–58.

20. Neimeyer RA, Keese B, Fortner M. Loss and meaning reconstruction: propositions and procedures. In: Malkinson R, Rubin S, Witztum E, eds. *Traumatic and Non-Traumatic Loss and Bereavement: Clinical Theory and Practice.* Madison, CT: International Universities Press; 2000: 197–230.

21. Neymeyer RA, Prigerson HG, Davies B. Mourning and meaning. *Am Behav Sci* 2002;46(2):235–51.

22. Klass D, Silverman P, Nickman S, eds. *Continuing Bonds: New Understandings of Grief.* Washington, DC: Taylor and Francis; 1996.

23. Prigerson HG, Maciejewski PK. A call for sound empirical testing and evaluation of criteria for complicated grief proposed for DSM-V. *Omega J Death Dying* 2005–2006;52(1):9–19.

24. Rubin S. A two-track model of bereavement: theory and research. *Am J Orthopsychiatry* 1981;51(1):101–9.

25. Rubin S, The two-track model of bereavement: overview, retrospect, and prospect. *Death Studies* 1999;23(8):681–714.

26. Bonanno GA. Loss, trauma, and human resilience: have we underestimated the human capacity to thrive after extremely adverse events? *Am Psychol* 2004;59:20–28.

27. Bonanno GA. *The Other Side of Sadness: What the New Science of Bereavement Tells Us about Life after a Loss.* New York: Basic Books; 2009.

28. Strada EA. Grief, demoralization, and depression: Diagnostic challenges and treatment modalities. *Primary Psychiatry* 2009;16(5):49–55.

Chapter 3

Cultural, Spiritual, and Developmental Aspects of Grief Reactions

Focus Points

- Patients' and caregivers' experience and expression of grief are shaped by many factors, including culture, community, stage of life, and spiritual and religious values.
- Clinicians are encouraged to approach every encounter with patients and caregivers as a "cross-cultural encounter" and to make an effort to understand the impact of cultural and spiritual/religious factors on grieving, avoiding preconceived notions and assumptions.
- Ability to recognize patients and caregivers' predominant grieving style will enable clinicians to more skillfully identify and meet grief and bereavement needs.

The ability to develop attachment to people, objects, places, and situations develops shortly after birth and remains a fundamental part of psychological functioning throughout life. And yet, the ability to form attachment is also a prerequisite for grief. Grief can be thought of as the reaction to the loss of what we have become attached to. A person's grief reaction to loss is deeply shaped by cultural, psychological, religious, and social variables. Therefore, clinicians should consider each patient and each caregiver as having not only an individual way or style to express grief but also an individual experience of grief. Developing the ability to recognize and support that unique expression is part of the mandate of palliative care clinicians, and it is an opportunity for other clinicians to deeply connect with the emotional realities of their patients.

Culture and Grief

Culture is a construct that encompasses language, beliefs, behaviors, social patterns, history, identity, and relationship with spiritual and religious beliefs.[1] Culture determines *what* can elicit a grief reaction, *how* grief should be expressed, *whether* it should be expressed, what normal expression of grief is, and what is against the norm. However, there is substantial variation within the same culture due to the modulating effects of personal and family history. Not only does grieving differ among cultures; it also differs among individuals within the same culture. And, to go even deeper, it often differs among members of the same family.

Because an attempt to understand someone's culture highlights the complexity of the construct, clinicians may find it tempting to rely on generalizations with the purpose of simplifying a challenging task. However, any simple or general statement about how people in a specific culture grieve may risk trivializing differences, oversimplifying the issues, and encouraging incorrect assumptions.[2] Clinicians will benefit from approaching patients and caregivers from cultures different from their own with complete openness and curiosity. Asking direct questions to patients and caregivers may be more effective and demonstrate the cultural sensitivity and cultural humility that is so important in palliative care. In the author's experience, patients and caregivers respond more favorably when clinicians ask them to describe their cultural practices and beliefs as they pertain to death and dying, rather than making incorrect assumptions based on generalizations.

General areas for exploration are as follows: (1) meaning of illness and death; (2) beliefs in afterlife; (3) acceptable and customary expressions of grief; (4) out of the ordinary or unacceptable expressions of grief; (5) cultural context of grief; and (6) relationship between private experience of grief and public manifestation (Table 3.1).

In most cases the experience and expression of grief are strongly influenced by the attachment styles in the family of origin and behaviors learned from

Table 3.1 Exploring Culturally Determined Aspects of Grief	
Meaning of illness and death	• Is there a concept of "good" or "bad" death? If so, how may it affect plan of care? • What is the explanation for the illness? • What is the explanation for the death? (punishment from God, etc.)
Beliefs in afterlife	• Does the relationship with deceased continue? Does the spirit of the decease return to visit the survivors? Does the death and dying process determine whether the spirit will be benevolent or angry?
Customary and pathological manifestations of grief	• Is grief acceptable only if expressed through physical symptoms? • Should grief be suppressed or expressed more prominently? • Do survivors feel supported or unsupported by prescribed cultural practices?
Internal and public expression of grief	• Does the culture encourage more (or less) public display as compared to the griever's internal experience of grief?
Sociocultural context of grief	• Are poverty, racism, and discrimination relevant to the cultural and personal grief narrative of the patient and the caregivers?

families and communities.[3,4] Borrowing from existential language, grieving can almost be thought of as *ways of being in the world after a loss*.

After the death of a loved one in the family, the adults generally model mourning practices for children. As a result, children learn what family and community consider adaptive ways of expressing grief.

For example, after a death in the family, the implicit message can be: "It is not ok to show too much distress and cry. It is not ok to put life on hold to grieve. Just keep it together, focus on getting things done, and look ahead." Or, the message can be completely different and encourage the expression of emotions and distress for prolonged periods of time. The cultural norms of a community may encourage suppression of strong affect as a way to exhibit control, dignity, and composure. Suppression of affect in certain circumstances can be adaptive and allow grievers to continue to perform tasks considered important at a time of crisis.

Other grievers do not intentionally suppress strong affect; simply, they do not experience grief as a devastating emotion and are able to continue on with life with relatively little distress. Assuming that these grievers were not attached to the loved one would be a mistake, based in old beliefs and biases about grief that are inconsistent with bereavement research. As mentioned in Chapter 2, while the early literature on bereavement identified strong expression of affect as the correct way of grieving, clinicians should remember that the evidence has shown that this is not the case. To add to the complexity, the grieving behaviors encouraged and developed in childhood, or from the first or most salient experiences of death, may or may not be an adequate match for the individual's character or predisposition. As a result, clinicians may encounter patients and caregivers with difficulty recognizing and expressing their grief in a manner that meets their needs.

The clinically meaningful question, therefore, isn't "Is the patient or caregiver grieving appropriately". Rather, it is: "Is the patient or caregiver expressing grief in a manner that is consistent with his or her personality style and cultural background, and is it supportive of the individual mourning process?"

Surprisingly, the extant literature lacks studies focused on identifying grieving styles in various populations of grievers. A model of adaptive grieving patterns was developed by Doka and Martin[5] and has been utilized as part of an Internet-based psychoeducation intervention to support normal grieving.[6] While more studies are needed to support the model, it will be briefly described here because of its relevance to clinical practice. Grieving styles are described along a continuum from intuitive to instrumental, and four patterns are identified: intuitive, instrumental, blended, and dissonant.

Intuitive grievers may experience grief as "waves" of feelings and may feel overwhelmed by the emotional pain of grief. They may display disorganized thinking, uncontrollable crying, and may benefit from being allowed to express their emotions. It is this author's experience that using the metaphor of ocean waves can resonate with these grievers, who may describe feeling as if they are literally drowning in pain. For this reason, the use of the ocean metaphor may validate the feeling of being overwhelmed by a "wave" of pain. The clinician may suggest that while the patient may feel in the middle of an ocean of despair and unable to see the shore, the shore is a reality. Encouraging the process, they can reassure that there is movement toward the shore, even though progress appears slows. Clinicians can then symbolically become holders of the hope that life will continue despite what feels to be devastating loss.

Instrumental grievers are primarily focused on problem solving and control over the environment. They may experience grief as a thought and be generally reluctant to talk about feelings. The ability to exhibit mastery of themselves and the environment is a core value. Obsessiveness, as well as confusion and forgetfulness, may be exhibited. Paradoxically they may experience a higher energy level than usual and engage in multiple activities. As a result, they may appear more productive and their internal grief may go unnoticed. Grievers who predominantly utilize this modality may be perceived as detached and disconnected from their grief, or at least as not needing support, which would be an incorrect assumption.

Dissonant grievers may express grief in one pattern but are, in fact, inhibited from finding ways to express grief that is compatible with their experience. This situation mostly occurs when intuitive grievers feel they cannot cry or express strong emotions. As a result, they express grief differently than they experience it and are caught in a serious emotional struggle. The grieving style model includes a blended pattern, where grievers utilize both intuitive (open expression of strong affect) and instrumental (grief primarily as an intellectual experience) strategies.

As mentioned earlier, the lack of empirical support for the grieving style model may limit its applicability and generalizability. However, it can provide clinicians with a good starting point in their efforts to explore patients and caregivers' unique way of experiencing and expressing grief (see Table 3.2).

Table 3.2 Grieving Styles	
Intuitive	• Grief experienced as waves of strong feelings
	• May experience periods of confusion, disorganization
	• May benefit from openly expressing grief
	• May express hopelessness, despair, suicidal ideation
Instrumental	• Grief experienced as a thought
	• May appear focused on control and "doing"
	• Grief reactions may go unnoticed
	• May not benefit from openly talking about loss
Dissonant	• Authentic grieving style may be suppressed
	• May react in ways that do not facilitate process
	• May be at risk for complicated grief
	• May benefit from psychological interventions
Source: Modified and adapted from Martin and Doka, 2010.	

The Culture of Grief in Families

Not uncommonly, members of the same family may approach grief and loss in different ways due to differences in personality and developmental stage; therefore, it is important to recognize and validate each person individually, as well as the family as a whole. Grieving styles within a family or a couple may be so different that communication difficulties and misunderstandings can occur and seriously undermine the ability to share and connect during palliative care and, subsequently, during bereavement. This potential "grieving mismatch" in couples and families represents another important area of assessment and intervention for trained clinicians.

Case Example

A young woman with metastatic ovarian cancer was admitted to the oncology floor and followed concurrently by palliative care. She immediately let everyone know that her main goal was to go home as soon as she was medically stable enough. Her husband and her parents were at the bedside around the clock. Her mother never left the hospital room and cried quietly most of the time; her father was primarily involved in making preparations for her return home. He would spend 10 minutes in the room and would then get up stating that he "needed to do something." He would check in with the nurses, make a phone call to update a family member, or get a glass of water for his wife, who kept asking him to sit with her. He would answer abruptly: "I am not going to just sit here and cry; that's useless." Unfortunately the patient continued to decline and it became apparent that she would not be able to be transferred home. She died a few days later. In the hours following her death, while she was still in the bed to allow for her loved ones to say good-bye, her father started pacing and anxiously asking various staff members: "What should I do? What should I do now? I don't know what I should do." He explained he needed "a task," something to do that would allow him to continue to move. He stated clearly he could not sit with his pain and cry, like his wife did. He found it impossible to sit with her and even hug her, as she asked him to do. He also stated he did not feel like crying in front of others because crying was "a private thing." His wife became even more distressed and blurted out, "What kind of man are you? Your daughter just died and you can't even cry? You can't even hug me and cry with me!" Her husband ignored her and repeated that he needed something to do. It became clear that each parent needed individualized support and help understanding the spouse's way of expressing grief. A family session provided a forum for expression of emotions and de-escalation of distress. Psychoeducation about different ways in which people grieve helped the wife understand her husband's behavior. Subsequently, members of the palliative care team sat with him helping him identify possible tasks. He started making a list of all the people who should be called and began leaving phone messages. He alternated this activity with checking in with his wife and going by his daughter's room to allow the reality of her death to slowly set in.

The main point to remember is that clinicians need to follow the insights and lead provided by patients and family members about their grieving needs, without inadvertently forcing a grieving style on them. Additionally, clinicians may need to function as "grief translators," facilitating communication between the grieving individual and others, who may misunderstand or negatively perceive what may actually be adaptive grieving behaviors.

Case Example

Anna was a 53-year-old retired physician and professor, diagnosed with advanced ovarian cancer. Chemotherapy treatment was initiated, but it was soon discontinued due to unmanageable side effects. Anna seemed to accept her diagnosis and poor prognosis in a very pragmatic way and announced to her family that while she felt very sad and did not want to leave them, she also felt peaceful and quite satisfied with her life and legacy as a physician and teacher. Anna was married, and she had two adult daughters and grandchildren. She did not express emotions openly and regarded crying as "understandable behavior, but essentially unproductive." When asked how she coped with her sadness, she commented that her grief was deep, but there was no point in focusing on it, because it would not change her situation.

Her daughters, on the other hand, felt devastated, cried constantly, and took leaves from their jobs, stating they wanted to spend as much time as possible with their mother. Anna's husband's grieving style was similar to his daughters; while Anna watched TV in her room he often sat with them in another room discussing their emotions. During an individual psychotherapy session, Anna commented feeling terribly sad about her poor prognosis, and she admitted often crying alone in her room, when no one would see her. She also commented she felt overwhelmed by her daughters' and husband's crying and felt she needed to protect herself from their emotional intensity. During a family session, her daughters and husband expressed feeling alone and isolated in their grief, and they stated it was as though Anna had already emotionally left them. Further exploration revealed Anna had been raised in a family that valued composure and suppression of emotions, especially in the face of adversity. While Anna pursued her medical career, her husband had been primary caregiver for their daughters, conveying to them the message that emotions should be openly expressed. It became clear that shared grief, instead of bring the family members closer, highlighted the different grieving cultures and fostered poor communication and hurt. Recognizing this reality allowed the family to accept therapeutic interventions to help develop a blended family grieving style that could honor different emotional needs.

Case Example

A young couple's baby was born prematurely and with a congenital heart defect deemed incompatible with survival. The baby spent over a month in intensive care. During that time several medical consultants visited, but it soon became apparent to the medical team that the baby was not going to survive. This was the young couple's first child and they were both very distressed.

During several meetings with the parents it became apparent that the inability to grieve together and support each other in their grieving process was causing additional distress. The mother was very expressive in her grief and felt the need to cry, to ask for help, and to surround herself with other women, family members, and friends, who would cry with her, sometimes physically hold her as she cried desperately. As she described it, she needed a "circle of support," where she could safely process her pain through crying and asking God for explanations. The husband, on the other hand, did not appear comfortable with such displays of strong emotions and became progressively detached from his wife. He started volunteering for extra shifts at work and began spending less time at home. His wife blamed him for "not being supportive" and complained that he did not cry, did not want to spend a lot of time talking about the baby, and did not share his emotions. He started experiencing severe low back pain and neck, shoulder pain, and frequent stomachaches. He stated that working more helped him "deal with it" and "feel less pain." His wife, however, was not feeling supported and believed that his pain was less intense. The mismatch in the grieving style resulted in inaccurate assumptions and serious marital conflict that seriously threatened this couples' ability to stay together in the midst of a tragic event.

These three cases illustrate a reality frequently observed in the palliative care setting: patients and caregivers may experience, process, and express their grief very differently. These differences may compromise their ability to be supportive of each other, which may be a risk factor for poor communication, sense of isolation, and conflict. Family members may not be aware of the existence of different styles within the same family. Psychoeducation is then an important intervention to prevent attributing behaviors to lack of love or lack of grief.

The focus on supporting individual expression of grief should not minimize the importance of monitoring and assessing for safety. However, recognition of at-risk behaviors may be a challenging task. For example, some patients and caregivers' expression of intense affect in public may not only be culturally acceptable but considered culturally and interpersonally necessary. Expression of strong affect, including incontrollable crying, yelling, and refusal to sleep, eat, or perform usual routines of self-care may be considered an appropriate demonstration of love for the patient. When rooted in cultural practices, these behaviors, which often have ritualistic value, are generally voluntarily stopped by the griever after what is considered an acceptable amount of time and may not be the expression of psychopathology. The challenge for palliative care and other clinicians is to differentiate among grief reactions that, while not mainstream, are culturally supported and therefore helpful to the griever, from uncontrollable expression of distress that requires professional help.

The Impact of Spirituality and Religion

Recognizing that spiritual and religious beliefs may have a strong impact on patients' and caregivers' ability to cope with loss, grief, and the death and

dying process, the Consensus Document for Quality Palliative Care identified spiritual and religious aspects of care as one of the domains of palliative
care.[7] Recent work has emphasized the importance for all palliative care clinicians to be aware of patients' and caregivers' personal preferences in this
area and have described specific guidelines for screening, assessment, and
intervention.[8,9]

Over the past decade, several studies have investigated the role of religion
and spirituality on patients' and caregivers' ability to cope with advanced illness, death, and bereavement. However, the existing literature highlights the
ongoing methodological challenges in this area, primarily related to how to
consistently operationalize and measure spiritual/religious concepts across
populations.

It has been proposed that religious beliefs are an integral part of the meaning-making process in bereavement. It has also been suggested that religious
affiliation can foster religious belonging, facilitating bereavement through rituals
and practices congruent with people's beliefs and existential values.[10,11] Studies
have also suggested that patients find their spiritual and religious beliefs help
them cope with their own illness, death, and dying.[12,14]

However, the relationship between religious coping and bereavement outcome variables, such as physical and psychological health, and adjustment level
is complex, and evidence from the literature is mixed.

Studies have found initial deterioration in physical well-being among people
who rely on religious beliefs to cope—also defined as "religious copers"—with
loss in the early stages of bereavement, but better functioning and decreased
disability months later.[13,16] Similarly, bereaved "religious copers" who had lost
a partner to AIDS reported more physical symptoms of acute grief in the
first month after death than people who did not rely on religion to cope with
bereavement.[17] Believing in the afterlife has been associated with less depressed
mood in bereaved parents of a child,[18] and strong spiritual or religious beliefs
and high levels of spiritual experience during church participation have also
been associated with better long-term overall adjustment.[22] However, "negative religious coping," characterized by spiritual struggle and anger at God, has
consistently been associated with worse physical health and quality of life, as
well as more depression in medically ill patients.[21] Additionally, mere church
attendance and religious participation without intrinsic faith belief were found
to have no impact on grief and depression[19] or was even associated with higher
levels of depression.[20–23]

While the lack of conclusive evidence from the literature confirms the
complexity of these issues, palliative care and other clinicians should approach
every patient as a unique individual and rely on screening, assessment, clinical
judgment, and interdisciplinary collaboration to determine the importance and
impact of spirituality and religion in each case. It should be emphasized that
chaplains are integral and invaluable members of the interdisciplinary health
care team and play a crucial role in assessing and addressing spiritual and
existential distress in patients and caregivers.[24]

When considering the impact of spirituality and religion on grief reactions, clinicians should remember the following:

- Strong spiritual/religious beliefs may help patients cope with preparatory grief from advanced illness and approaching death, and they may similarly help caregivers before and during bereavement.
- Simply belonging to a religious organization or attending service does not automatically translate into improved ability to cope with grief, death and dying, and bereavement.
- Instead of assuming that spiritual orientation and/or religious affiliation is a protective factor and a source of support, palliative care clinicians should gently explore whether patients' and caregivers' beliefs are a *current* and *active* source of strength and support.
- Palliative care clinicians should also listen for any expression of spiritual or religious struggle and suffering, which may need to be addressed by a professional spiritual care provider.

Developmental Aspects of Grief and Bereavement

Grief and bereavement care in the palliative setting includes the family and other caregivers, presenting clinicians with the challenge of providing support to several different people who may be at very different developmental stages. Grandparents and other older adults, as well as children, may be part of the network of caregivers around the patient. Different life stages often translate into different ways of processing death and grief. Therefore, recognizing variations in the expression of grief across the life span can help palliative care clinicians provide the sensitive, age-appropriate, and individualized support that can more effectively relieve suffering.

Grief Reactions in Children and Adolescents

Children are a constant part of the family system and network of caregiving around palliative care patients. They often accompany adult members and other caregivers to the hospital to visit their parents, grandparents, and other relatives with advanced illness. Even though there is usually an adult present, clinicians should not assume that children's grief reactions are always recognized and supported, especially when the adult caregivers are already feeling overwhelmed. Therefore, clinicians should be at least aware of general developmental issues that affect children's understanding of death and their experience and expression of grief.

It is important that grief and bereavement care in the palliative care and hospice setting should extend to children and adolescents, so they will feel included and reassured.[25,26]

Children's experience grief and emotional distress may be profound. However, depending on their developmental stage and level of language acquisition, they may not be able to verbally communicate, show, or articulate their pain as openly as adults can do. Children, especially very young ones, are more likely to express their feeling through behaviors, rather than through verbal communication. Most important, children's reaction to loss is significantly impacted by the way family members react to the loss. Even very young children are able to detect subtle messages communicated by the family and the groups surrounding.[27]

Infants are obviously unable to understand the concept of death, but they can be deeply affected by the loss of primary caregiver and may react with profound distress to the loss of attachment figures. They may display uncontrollable crying, lack of sleep, weight loss, and become apathetic. The core issues that need addressing are safety and attachment. Maintaining routines while providing physical and verbal reassurance can be a helpful intervention.[28]

Between the ages of 2 and 3, children are still unable to cognitively understand the concept of death, but they are profoundly affected by the loss of a primary attachment figure. They may express grief through prolonged emotional and social withdrawal, as well as changes in eating and sleeping pattern. They may also display regressive behaviors and temporary loss of previously acquired abilities and skills.[29] Maintaining routines and providing physical and emotional reassurance and support are important. Rather than constantly hiding their own grief, adults can provide simple explanations for their emotions. Maintaining routines can be especially difficult for the surviving spouse when there is loss of a parent. Therefore, clinicians should not assume that parents will automatically be able to care for their children in the early phases of grief after losing a spouse. Practical help from family members and friends can be especially helpful in maintaining a sense of structure and routine that may reassure the child, increasing a sense of safety and continuity.

Between the ages of 3 and 6, children think in concrete ways and may not be able to understand that death is a permanent condition. They are still unable to fully understand the difference between life and death and may think that someone who has died is sleeping or that he or she is away on a trip and may come back at some point. Children at this stage of development often use magical thinking in their way of understanding the world and relating to it.[30] This knowledge has important clinical implications in the palliative care setting, where family members often ask providers for guidance about the appropriate way to talk to children about a loved one who is dying.

Between the ages of 6 and 9, children are still thinking concretely but may be able to understand that death is a physical phenomenon. However, they may think that the loved one continues to live somewhere else as they may not be able to fully comprehend the permanency of death. Magical thinking is affected by the need for mastery that is typical of this developmental stage. As a result, they may think that angry thoughts about a loved one can cause sickness and death. These beliefs can generate profound guilt and anxiety in a child. Children at this stage may also display "acting out" behaviors as manifestations of grief. For example, they may become afraid of going to school, may become aggressive toward adults and other children, or may develop anxious preoccupations about their health and their body.[31]

Between the ages of 9 and 12, children undergo a significant level of cognitive and emotional development. By age 12, children are able to understand that death is a permanent condition and it happens to everyone. Because of their increased ability to feel complex emotions, they are at higher risk for becoming depressed or anxious, developing conduct problems, and may require assessment for professional help.[32]

Adolescents' grief reactions are often deeply affected by their need to be accepted by peers. As a result, they may resist the overt expression of emotions during the grieving process, for fear of being considered weak by the peer group. The adolescent who would feel inclined to express strong emotions, but feels inhibited doing so out of fear, shame, or due to lack of supportive community, may feel metaphorically "trapped" and engage in aggressive or self-disruptive behaviors as outlets for expression of painful emotions. Family dynamics may also present risk factors for bereaved adolescents. Grieving parents who feel emotionally overwhelmed may underestimate the adolescent's grieving process, or they may believe they are "grown-ups" and can handle their grief. Even though adolescents understand fully the meaning of death, they may display behaviors indicative of denial and are at high risk for maladaptive coping behaviors, such as alcohol and substance use, reckless driving, or violent acting out.[33]

Grief Reactions in Older Adults

Older adults represent a vulnerable population that can be particularly affected by grief reactions, especially because they may not be able to access resources typically available to younger people. Aging itself is a process that may involve grief, due to the systematic and progressive losses involved. Some of the losses are primary and concrete losses, such as the sensory and psychomotor changes that become common as people age, or the deaths of family members and friends. In addition, there are symbolic losses, such as loss of status and identity that can often accompany retirement.[34-40] Overall, aging involves multiple changes that impact on physical, psychological, and spiritual domains. Changes can be perceived as sudden and traumatic; others are subtler and occur over a period of time, thus allowing the psyche to adapt to a new psychophysical reality. Aging may also bring the awareness of mortality closer to daily life. Awareness that the amount of time one has to live is substantially less than the time one has already lived may cause psychological and existential suffering, especially if patients are experiencing regret about the past. Older people are at significant risk for experiencing bereavement overload; the losses may become so frequent that they can no longer be processed and integrated. As a result, each new loss adds to the distress already present, with the potential of engendering hopelessness and despair.

While acquired experience and wisdom can help balance the difficulty adjusting to the losses involved in the aging process, including the awareness that death may be near, the challenges faced by the elderly who are also dealing with end-of-life issues should not be minimized.

Older patients with advanced illness face unique challenges as they physically decline and approach the end of life. Patients may experience several comorbid conditions, including high levels of emotional distress, which can complicate the clinical presentation. There should be a low threshold for obtaining a thorough grief and bereavement assessment with this particularly vulnerable population. It may reveal the presence of grief reactions related to the aging process, to the dying process, and issues that are at the interface of aging and dying. For example, psychological difficulties experienced by patients adjusting to the loss of physical function, social roles, and personal identity due to the aging process should be addressed therapeutically, and they may need to be differentiated from the preparatory grief experienced by patients who are dying.[41–50] Older bereaved caregivers are at higher risk for complicated grief, depression, and anxiety.[51] Additionally, bereaved grandparents may experience what has been described as "double pain," which means they experience grief for the death of a grandchild and grief for their own child's loss.[52] It is undeniable that older bereaved caregivers and older patients face numerous challenges as they face bereavement and advanced illness. Often, their grief goes unrecognized and may become disenfranchised. It is crucial that clinicians in the palliative care and hospice setting recognize the risks in this vulnerable population and address them accordingly.

References

1. Carrillot JE, Green AR, Betancourt JR. Cross-cultural primary care: a patient-based approach. *Ann Int Med* 1999;130(10):829–34.

2. Rosenblatt PC. Cross-cultural variation in the experience, expression, and understanding of grief. In: Irish DP, Lundy KF, Nelsen VJ, eds. *Ethnic Variations in Dying, Death and Grief: Diversity in Universality*. Washington, DC: Taylor & Francis; 1993:13–19.

3. Mikulincer M, Shaver PR, Pereg D. Attachment theory and affect regulation: the dynamics, development, and cognitive consequences of attachment-related strategies. *Motivation Emotions* 2003;27(2):77–102.

4. Kalish R, Reynolds D. *Death and Ethnicity: A Psychocultural Study*. Los Angeles, CA: University of California Press; 1976.

5. Doka KJ, Martin TL. *Grieving Beyond Gender: Understanding the Ways Men and Women Mourn*. New York: Routledge; 2010.

6. Dominick SA, Irvine AB, Beauchamp N, et al. An internet tool to normalize grief. *Omega* 2009;60(1):71–87.

7. National Consensus Project for Quality Palliative Care. Clinical Practice Guidelines for Quality Palliative Care. 2004, Brooklyn, NY: National Consensus Project for Quality Palliative Care.

8. Puchalski C, Ferrell BR, Virani R, et al. Improving the quality of spiritual care as a dimension of palliative care: the report of the consensus conference. *J Palliat Med* 2009;12(10):885–904.

9. Puchalsky CM, Ferrell B. *Making Healthcare Whole: Integrating Spirituality into Patient Care*. West Conshohocken, PA: Templeton Press; 2010.

10. Barbour IG. *Religion in an Age of Science: The Gifford Lectures 1989–1991. Vol. 1.* San Francisco, CA: Harper & Row; 1990.

11. Bergin AE. Values and religious issues in psychotherapy and mental health. *Am Psychol* 1991;46:394–403.

12. Bergin AE, Strupp HH. *Changing Frontiers in the Science of Psychotherapy.* Chicago, IL: Aldine; 1972.

13. Ano GG, Vasconcelles EB. Religious coping and psychological adjustment to stress: a meta-analysis. *J Clin Psychol* 2005;61:461–80.

14. Alcorn SR, Balboni MJ, Prigerson HG, et al. If God wanted me yesterday, I wouldn't be here today: Religious and spiritual themes in patients' experiences of advanced cancer. *J Palliative Med* 2010;13(5):581–8.

15. Breitbart W. Spirituality and meaning in supportive care: spirituality and meaning-centered group psychotherapy interventions in advanced cancer. *Support Care Cancer* 2002;10:272–80.

16. Pearce MJ, Chen J, Silverman GK, et al. Religious coping, health, and health service use among bereaved adults. *Intl J Psychiatry Med* 2002;32:179–99.

17. Richards TA, Folkman S. Spiritual aspects of loss at the time of a partner's death from AIDS. *Death Studies* 1997;21:527–52.

18. Higgins MP. Parental bereavement and religious factors. *Omega: J Death Dying* 2002;45:187–207.

19. Abrums M. Death and meaning in a storefront church. *Pub Health Nursing* 2000;17:132–42.

20. Austin D, Lennings CJ. Grief and religious beliefs: does belief moderate depression? *Death Studies* 1993;17:487–96.

21. Koenig HG, Pargament KI, & Nielsen J. Religious coping and health status in medically ill hospitalized older adults. *Journal of Nervous and Mental Disease,* 1998;186:153–521., ed. *Handbook of Religion and Mental Health.* San Diego, CA: Academic Press; 1998.

22. Easterling LW, Gamino LA, Sewell KW, Stirman LS. Spiritual experience, church attendance, and bereavement. *J Pastoral Care* 2000;54:267–75.

23. Rosik CH. The impact of religious orientation in conjugal bereavement among older adults. *Intl J Aging Human Dev* 1989;28:251–60.

24. Cooper RS. Case Study of a Chaplain's Spiritual Care for a Patient with Advanced Metastatic Breast Cancer. *J Health Care Chaplain* 2011;17(1):19–37.

25. Librach SL, O'Brien H. Supporting children's grief within an adult and pediatric palliative care program. *J Support Oncol* 2011;9(4):136–40.

26. Torbic H. Children and grief: but what about the children? A guide for home care and hospice clinicians. *Home Health Nurse* 2011;29(2):67–77.

27. Reeves N. *A Path Tthrough Loss.* Victoria, BC: Northstone; 2001.

28. Slaughter V. Young children understanding of death. *Australian Psychol* 2005;40(3):179–86.

29. Doka KJ. *Children Mourning, Mourning Cchildren.* New York: Routledge; 1995.

30. Silverman PR & Kelly M. *A Parent's Guide to Raising Grieving Children: Rebuilding Your Family after the Death of a Loved One.* New York: Oxford; 2009.

31. Wolfelt AD. *Healing a Child's Grieving Heart: 100 Practical Ideas for Families, Friends, and Caregivers.* Fort Collins, CO: Companion Press; 2001.

32. Webb NB. *Helping Bereaved Children: A Handbook for Practitioners.* New York: Guilford Press; 2010.

33. Balk D. Adolescents' grief reactions and self-concept perception following sibling death- a study of 33 teenagers. *J Youth Adolescence* 1983;12(2):137–67.

34. Birren JE, Fisher LM. Aging and speed behavior: possible consequences for psychological functioning. *Ann Rev Psychol* 1995;46:329–53.

35. De la Fuente M. Effects of antioxidants on immune system ageing. *Eur J ClinNutr* 2002;56(3):S5.

36. Dowd JJ. *Stratification Among the Aged.* Monterey, CA: Brooks Cole; 1980.

37. Ellerman CR, Reed PG. Self-transcendence and depression in middle age adults. *West J Nurs Res* 2001;23(7):698.

38. Erikson EH, Erikson JM, Kivnick HQ. *Vital Involvement in Old Age: The Experience of Old Age in Our Time.* New York: Norton; 1986.

39. Hayflick L. *How and Why We Age.* New York: Ballantine Books; 1996.

40. Knight BG, McCallum TJ. Adapting psychotherapeutic practice for older clients: implications of the contextual, cohort-based, maturity, specific challenge model. *Prof Psychol Res Practice* 1998;29:15–22.

41. Hatch LR. Gender and ageism. *Generations* 2005;29:19–25.

42. Havighurst RJ, Neugarten BL, Tobin SS. Disengagement and patterns of aging. In: Neugarten BL (ed.) *Middle Age and Aging: A Reader in Social Psychology.* Chicago, IL: University of Chicago Press; 1968:223–237.

43. Herth, K. Fostering hope in terminally-ill people. *J Adv Nurs* 1990;15:1250–9.

44. Hooks, B. *Feminist Theory: From Margin to Center.* Cambridge, MA: South End Press; 2000.

45. Hooyman NR, Kiyak HA. *Social Gerontology: A Multidisciplinary Perspective.* 7th ed. New York: Pearson; 2005.

46. Jett KF. The meaning of aging and the celebration of years among rural African-American women. *Geriatric Nurs* 2003;24(5):290.

47. Jung CG. The stages of life. In Campbell J, ed. *The Portable Jung.* New York: Viking Press; 1971:163–177.

48. Karier CJ. *Scientists of the Mind: Intellectual Founders of Modern Psychology.* Chicago, IL: University of Illinois Press; 1986.

49. La Rue A, Watson J. (1998). Psychological assessment of older adults. *Prof Psychol Res Practice* 1998;29:5–14.

50. Szanto K, Gildengers A, Mulsant BH, Brown G, Alexopoulos GS, Reynolds CF, 3rd. Identification of suicidal ideation and prevention of suicidal behaviour in the elderly. *Drugs Aging* 2002;19(1):11–24.

51. Newson RS, Boelen PA, Hek K, Hofman A, Tiemeier H. The prevalence and characteristics of complicated grief in older adults. *J Affect Disord* 2011;132(1–2):231–8.

52. Gilrane-McGarry U, Grady T. Forgotten grievers: an exploration of the grief experience of bereaved grandparents. *Int J Palliat Nurs* 2011;17(4):170–6.

Chapter 4

Normal Grief, Anticipatory Grief, and Complicated Grief

Focus Points

- In patients and caregivers, normal grief can be associated with significant physical, emotional, and spiritual distress that can last for variable periods of time.
- Anticipatory (preparatory) grief can be experienced by patients who are approaching death and caregivers who care for them before the actual death. Preparatory grief in patients with advanced illness is not a pathological process, but it involves a complex and sometimes distressing process of adjustment to progressing illness and approaching death.
- Complicated grief is a form of unresolved grief resulting in persistent and disabling pathology, which warrants psychological and medical evaluation and treatment. While mostly studied in reference to bereaved caregivers, complicated grief can also be experienced patients with advanced illness.

Depending on the setting, phenomenology, and clinical manifestations, grief has been divided into different categories. It could be argued that describing grief subtypes is somewhat artificial and using different terms to describe it does not essentially change the constellation of symptoms experienced by grievers. However, while the core of the grief experience may be substantially similar, the implications of the various grief reactions often raise different concerns and risk factors, which need to be appropriately addressed by palliative care and other clinicians.

Normal Grief after the Death of Someone Close

In bereavement, *normal grief*, or nonpathological grief, refers to the physical and emotional reactions that can be experienced after the death of someone close. While the term is commonly used to refer to the natural response to loss, normal grief has the potential to cause significant impairment and disability. Clinicians should remember that, even if grief is normal, it may feel far from normal to the patient or caregiver who is experiencing it. The effects of normal grief vary in duration and intensity, affecting individuals on a physical, psychological, cognitive, and spiritual level, and can cause significant suffering for prolonged periods of time.[1-3] Along these lines, it is not uncommon for bereaved individuals to make statements such as "I feel like I am losing my mind"; "I have no control over anything"; "I think I am going crazy"; "My entire body hurts— something must be seriously wrong."

Because symptom burden and distress in the early phases of bereavement can present with the same intensity as in complicated grief, predicting the course can be challenging.

For many survivors, bereavement may involve an initial period of shock, disbelief, or denial. Others may immediately start suffering from physical, emotional, cognitive, behavioral, and spiritual distress. Physical reactions to loss may include shortness of breath, tightness in the throat, feeling of emptiness and heaviness, physical numbness, feeling outside one's body, muscle tension, body aches, headaches, dizziness, nausea, gastrointestinal problems, and heart palpitations. Commonly experienced are also somatic symptoms of depression, such as crying spells, fatigue, sleep disturbances, anorexia, weight loss, lack of strength, loss of sexual desire, or hypersexualiy.[4-10]

Normal grief can also include temporary perceptual disturbances, such as visual and auditory hallucinations; impaired memory; constant worry; slowed and disorganized thinking; suicidal ideation; and constant preoccupation with the deceased.[11,12] The content of the perceptual disturbances is often related to difficult or traumatic circumstances surrounding the death of the person who died, or unresolved issues that may elicit guilt. For example, caregivers who have cared for someone one who experienced unmanaged pain at the end of life may report continuing to hear the loved one call out in pain. Similarly, caregivers whose family members experienced poorly managed agitated terminal delirium may report nightmares and intrusive memories of the traumatic experience, especially if the images of distress and agitation are their last memory.[13,14] Caregivers who have felt helpless witnessing physical or emotional suffering at the end of life may continue to experience a sense of helplessness, guilt, resentment, and anger.

Normal grief can also affect neuroendocrine and immune function and sleep patterns.[15-18] In particular, studies have shown that in the early stages of bereavement there may be a cortisol response, immune imbalance due to reduced T-lymphocyte proliferation, changes in heart rate and blood pressure, and increased inflammation response.[54-56] Overall, bereaved individuals are at higher risk for morbidity and death.[57] Table 4.1 lists several reactions that can be experienced in the course of normal grief.

While the protective value of spirituality and religion in bereavement has been generally supported,[19,20] some bereaved individuals may develop doubts in faith beliefs, especially after traumatic deaths. Grief can trigger spiritual distress, which may manifest with conflicts in faith beliefs and loss of meaning and purpose. For this reason, clinicians should not necessarily assume that spiritual and religious affiliation is always a protective factor. Individual assessment of the patients and family may indicate the need for further explorations of spiritual issues with the help of a professional spiritual care provider.

In normal grief, acute symptoms tend to diminish in frequency and intensity over time, allowing for integration of the loss and continuation of daily

Table 4.1 Manifestations of Normal Grief

Physical	Emotional	Cognitive	Behavioral	Spiritual
Gastrointestinal disturbances	Helplessness	Disbelief	Withdrawal	Conflict in faith beliefs
Heart palpitations	Hopelessness	Depersonalization	Social isolation	Loss of meaning
Tightness in the chest	Anxiety	Lack of concentration	Avoidance	Spiritual suffering
Breathlessness	Depression	Confusion	Risk-taking behaviors	Hopelessness
Lack of energy	Despair	Fleeting tactile, visual, auditory hallucinatory experiences	Increased alcohol use	
Dry mouth	Anger	Memory impairment	Suicidal thoughts	
Loss of libido	Shock	Disturbing dreams		
Appetite changes	Relief			
Dizziness	Guilt			
Weight changes	Shame			
Sleep problems	Yearning			

functioning. The length of time necessary for the loss to be processed and integrated, which is usually referred to in the literature as a period of "restitution" is, however, variable, unique to the individual, and often unpredictable.[21] Even in the context of normal grief, those at high risk may need further medical and psychological evaluation and treatment, including short-term use of medication to improve sleep or decrease severe and disabling anxiety. Bereaved individuals with preexisting medical conditions may need to be evaluated by their primary care physician to rule out medical complications. These issues are further discussed in Chapter 5.

Variables Affecting the Course of Normal Grief

The course of normal grief in bereavement is affected by a number of variables, such as the survivor's relationship to the deceased, the survivor's level of functioning and mental health prior to the loss, and the nature and circumstances of the death.[22,23] These variables or factors may facilitate normal grieving, or they may interfere with it. Additionally, the impact of the various factors needs to be evaluated in the context of protective elements that can minimize risk, such as availability of social support before and after the death. Nonetheless, all the variables have to be carefully considered by clinicians during the assessment phase, because they may represent risk factors for complicated grief (see Table 4.2).

Table 4.2 Identifying Variables Influencing Caregivers' Grieving Process

Circumstances of the death
- Was the death sudden and unexpected?
- How long was the illness before the death?
- Do caregivers feel that the death could have been prevented?
- What was the general psycho-social-spiritual context before and after the death?

Relationship between the patient and caregivers before and during the illness
- Was there ambivalence in the relationship?
- Were there unresolved issues between the patient and the caregivers?
- Was there a history of abuse or addiction in the family, and how was that integrated in the family dynamics?
- Was the primary caregiver so dependent on the patient that he or she cannot imagine being able to function after the death?

Personal characteristics of the caregiver
- Did the caregiver experience other significant losses in the recent past?
- Was the caregiver already suffering from complicated grief for past unprocessed losses?
- What are the current/concurrent stressors for the caregiver?
- Does the caregiver have a history of mental health problems?
- What is the caregiver's developmental stage (child, adolescent, young adult, elderly) and how does it affect the reaction to the death?
- What are relevant cultural, ethnic, and spiritual variables that affect the caregiver's grieving process?

Anticipatory (Preparatory) Grief in Family Caregivers

The term *anticipatory grief* has been commonly used in the literature to describe the range of grief reactions occurring in family caregivers prior to the actual death of a loved one,[24–27] when the death is expected. It was originally used by Lindemann[24] to refer to the absence of overt manifestations of grief at the actual time of death by survivors who had already experienced symptoms of acute grief before the death. According to his description, intense grieving prior to the actual death allowed survivors to better manage post-death bereavement. The evidence from the literature about the nature and impact of anticipatory grief is inconsistent. Some researchers have contended that anticipatory grief is not a real phenomenon and is often confused with forewarning of death; other studies have argued the positive impact of anticipatory grief on post-death bereavement; yet others have shown that anticipatory grieving has a negative impact on bereavement. See Reynolds and Botha, 2006[28] for a review. While there is still significant debate around it, it is utilized as a framework for understanding caregiver's experiences in the palliative care setting.[29–34] The transition to palliative care can elicit significant anticipatory grief not only in patients, but also in caregivers, who may experience sadness, anger, and helplessness.[35,53] Therefore, it is crucial to include caregivers and their anticipatory grieving process in the care plan. Clinicians should remember that, while palliative care can significantly improve patients' quality of life, patients and caregivers may need a great deal of support from the team to adjust to the new reality of care and its implications.[36,37] Difficult transitions of care and a prolonged illness can elicit profound grief reactions, which can be especially prominent when the illness itself causes a change in the relationship, such as in patients with dementia.[38,39] Moreover, a combination of anticipatory grief and ambiguous loss has been found to represent a significant barrier to the task of caregiving.[40] While a certain degree of active grieving and distress in caregivers prior to the death of the loved one is normal and should be expected, clinicians should not underestimate its impact. When anticipatory grief is manageable, the level of distress fluctuates, allowing for valuable moments of peaceful emotional connection between caregivers and patients. However, for some caregivers anticipatory grief may represent a serious challenge. A Swedish study showed that four out of ten widows considered the period before the death of the spouse worse than bereavement.[41] The experience of caregivers of patients with lung cancer was described as centered on transition, with caregivers expressing a strong need for stability.[42] A study of Chinese, European Americans, Japanese, and Native Hawaiians caregivers showed that, while participants in the different cultural groups processed grief differently, they described similar stressors in caregiving and anticipatory grieving.[43] Severe and constant levels of anticipatory grief may elicit an acute grief reaction in the caregivers, as if the death had already occurred. As a result, there may be an emotional disconnect from the family member still alive with avoidant behavior, confusion, sense of abandonment, and suffering.

Family members and other caregivers who exhibit high levels of anticipatory grief should be identified by the palliative care team and receive a thorough grief and bereavement assessment. Caregivers who share with the team suicidal thoughts as a contingency plan for after the death should become a priority.[44] Psychological support should be considered to minimize the risk of complicated grief after the death. However, referring high-risk family members for grief counseling or therapy may be challenging. In many cases, caregivers are busy at work during the day and may visit the patient at the hospital during the afternoon or evening. They may recognize the need for psychological help, but they may lack the emotional energy or motivation to visit a mental health professional. Thus, whenever possible, palliative care clinicians should be able to provide interventions to family members in the hospital setting, during their visits.

Anticipatory (Preparatory) Grief in Patients with Advanced Illness

The grief experience of patients with advanced illness should be carefully understood, assessed, and supported, because it presents unique features that warrant an individualized approach.[45,64] In addition to anticipatory, the term *preparatory grief* has been used in the literature to indicate the normal grieving process experienced by patients with advanced illness as they approach death.[36,37,46,47] It may involve intense psychological work necessary to process grief about past, current, and anticipated physical and symbolic losses. Its presence and manifestation is strongly influenced by patients' demographics as well as past medical history.[48] Spiritual orientation and religious beliefs modulate the extent to which the patient's own death is perceived as an absolute loss of self or a transition to another existence of self that is primarily spiritual.

Preparatory grief has been described as a natural element of the life cycle,[46] with the potential of creating significant suffering for the patient and the family system. Kubler-Ross described preparatory grief as the grief that "the terminally ill patient has to undergo to prepare himself for his final separation from this world."[49] Patients who never use the word "death" or "dying," or never explicitly acknowledge awareness of approaching death may nonetheless experience variable degrees of preparatory grief.

Presence of preparatory grief in patients with advanced illness is not a sign of psychopathology, but a normal response to the inevitable and progressive losses they are facing individually as well as members of their family and their community.[50] However, in the same way normal grief in bereavement can sometimes turn into a pathological reaction, patients' preparatory grief can trigger or worsen depression and severe anxiety or become otherwise unmanageable.[52] Anxiety has been identified as the strongest clinical predictor of high levels of preparatory grief, followed by hopelessness, preexisting depression, and awareness of metastatic disease in patients with cancer.[37] Consistent with these results, levels of traumatic distress, in particular avoidance, intrusion, and

hyperarousal have been found to be highly correlated with high levels of preparatory grief.[47] Additionally, preparatory grief and depression were found to be
predictors of global hopelessness.

The Challenges of Patients' Preparatory Grief

Each patient's experience of preparatory grief is unique and no single framework can capture its complexity. It is important to clarify that patients with
advanced illness do not necessarily need to be engaged in any type of psychological work and clinicians should never impose on patients their own concept
of what death and dying should look like. However, it could be argued that,
along their journey through illness, including end of life, patients face a number of psychological, existential, and spiritual challenges that may affect their
experience and manifestation of preparatory grief. Examples of challenges that
patients may experience are briefly described below.

Awareness of Prognosis

One challenge involves dealing with the reality of a limited prognosis and progressive illness that will likely cause death. Every patient approaches this aspect
in unique ways. For example, patients at some level may have awareness that
death may be close, but they may choose to never openly acknowledge it with
caregivers or clinicians. Patients may hold hope for a miracle and awareness
that they are dying at the same time and may choose not to commit to any one
outcome. They may speak about their prognosis intentionally using ambiguous
metaphors that allow them to protect their psyche from facing the thought of
the inevitability of their death. In other words, patients often display what I call
"self-directed awareness and acceptance," which may help them maintain a certain sense of control and have adaptive value. While bereaved family members
are faced with the challenge of accepting that the loved one is, in fact, dead,
and no longer living, patients may experience various degrees of awareness
and acceptance of the fact that their death is near. Their willingness to openly
acknowledge that they are dying should not necessarily be interpreted as a sign
of benign acceptance and "better" adjustment to the dying process, the same
way that unwillingness to openly acknowledge that death is near is not necessarily a sign of unhealthy denial. Open awareness of dying does not automatically translate into acceptance or peace. Similarly, while patients may choose
not to openly acknowledge they are dying, they may still be internally engaged
in processing this reality.

Death awareness is a complex construct, initially explored in Glaser and
Straus's landmark study Awareness of Dying,[51] which described possible scenarios reflective of awareness contexts between patients and caregivers.
The types of awareness described in their study are (1) open, (2) suspected,
(3) mutual pretense, and (4) closed. In open awareness both patient and caregiver are aware that the patient is dying and can openly talk about it. In closed
awareness the caregiver is aware that the patient is dying, but this awareness

is hidden from the patient, with the intention of protecting the patient from emotional distress. In suspected awareness the patient suspects, but the topic is not openly discussed. Each person is focused on protecting the other from distress. In mutual pretense one or both parties in the patient–caregiver dyad pretend that they do not know the patient is dying. Many factors impact how awareness of dying is conceptualized by patients and caregivers. Cultural, spiritual, and religious beliefs, and family history, including perceived ability of the patient or caregiver's ability to cope with the impending death are some of the factors that add to the complexity of the issue. Palliative care clinicians must recognize that different ways of processing awareness of advanced illness, poor prognosis, and approaching death will affect the patient, family caregivers, and their relationship to each other in profound ways. It is important that personal styles and preferences be respected, without attempting to impose a modality that may not be recognized as valuable by patient and family. At times, palliative care clinicians may observe that previously adaptive communication styles in the family may no longer be supportive of patients' goals. For example, a patient's desire to openly discuss their approaching death and related grief may elicit fear and overwhelming grief in family members who may feel unprepared for an open conversation. They may attempt to avoid the subject by minimizing the seriousness of the patient's illness and providing superficial reassurance. As a result, the relationship between the patient and family members can become strained and emotional disconnect may ensue. In these and similar cases, palliative care clinicians can play an important role gently exploring patients' and families' concerns and help facilitate expression and processing of grief.

Transitions of Care

Transition from a curative to a palliative modality of care may also present a significant emotional challenge. As mentioned previously in reference to anticipatory grief in caregivers, transition to palliative care has often prognostic implications. The care provided by the palliative care team aims to allow patients the best quality of life possible for as long as they can. However, even the best palliative care cannot prevent patients from feeling profound grief, once they may realize that their journey through illness has taken on a completely different path from the one they wished for. Grief reactions to transitions of care should not be ignored or bypassed, but recognized and supported.

Fluctuating Level of Engagement

Another significant challenge many patients face is the need to modulate their level of physical and emotional engagement with their loved ones and the outside world, as they continue to decline. It is possible that the progressive emotional withdrawal that many patients experience as they approach death may be caused not only by the physical and cognitive decline but also by a progressive grieving process that facilitates patients' symbolic disinvestment of emotional energy from the world. Not all patients actively process the idea of separation from the world and loved ones. However, many patients may start imagining what their family will be like after their death, and they may benefit from help imagining a situation where the family is cared for. However, at this stage patients may express ambivalence as part of the grieving process. One patient commented, "My wife and my children keep telling I don't have to worry about them. They keep telling me that they will be ok and that I can be at peace. They are trying to help. I would never tell them this, but I am tired of hearing that they will be fine. I want them to be fine, but I want them to miss me and, in some way, not to be fine. But I love them and I want them to be fine! And this is the most painful thing for me" (verbatim from a recorded psychotherapy session).

Not uncommonly, patients face the challenge of finding a way to maintain a sense of meaningful connection with their loved ones in the context of the relationship and shared history, which transcends death. Patients may use various strategies in this process. Some may rely on their spiritual and religious beliefs. During family and couple's therapy sessions I have heard patients and family members negotiate their enduring connections, by saying, "I will always be close to you and pray for you and protect you" or "If there is another reality after death I will find a way to let you know I am fine and will watch over you." In many cases, palliative care clinicians are witnesses of this naturally unfolding process and shared grief.[64]

However, one assessment element to consider is that any strategy used to ensure enduring connections should be beneficial both to the patient and caregivers. Patients may make requests that can be distressing for family members: for example, asking a surviving spouse to never remarry so the connection will continue; asking children to promise they will choose a specific career path or to promise they will never marry someone the patient did not approve of; asking family members to promise they will never speak to someone the patient is upset with. There may be circumstances where these requests are acceptable to the family and do not cause emotional burden. However, some caregivers may find them distressing, and this may complicate their grieving process. Palliative care clinicians may want to be aware of these issues and gently explore their meaning with the patient and caregivers. Overall, the task for the palliative care team is to understand and facilitate dying patients' grieving process, as well as guiding and supporting the family. It needs to be emphasized that, in the context of palliative care patients, the challenges of preparatory grief are not to be understood as linear, sequential, or explicit. As mentioned earlier, each patient follows a unique process of adaptation and adjustment to advanced illness. However, clinicians may find it useful to keep these challenges in mind as a general guideline to identify areas that are the focus of the patient's grieving energy.

Complicated Grief (AKA Prolonged Grief Disorder)

In the last decade, the grief and bereavement literature has been impacted by an increasing amount of research, which has primarily focused on improving understanding of pathological grief reactions. Even though the majority of bereaved individuals are able to integrate the loss of someone close after a variable period of time, in 10% to 25% of cases bereaved individuals continue to experience distress so severe that it significantly impairs functioning and often precipitates psychiatric disorders such as major depression and anxiety disorders.[58–60]

Complicated grief, also called prolonged grief disorder, indicates a grieving process that does not move forward, where the griever is overwhelmed, unable to integrate the loss and adjust to it, even after long periods of prolonged distress.[61–63] In normal grief the intensity of distress fluctuates and slowly and gradually diminishes, allowing the griever to integrate the loss over time. The process of adaptation in normal grief is painful and slow; however, the majority of individuals, with enough support, do adjust. Generally, after 6–12 months the majority of bereaved individuals can adjust to the reality of the loss and find a way of continuing living a meaningful life. To suggest that in normal grief "things go back to normal" would be inappropriate and clinically contraindicated, because a major loss changes the griever in profound ways. And, while in many cases grievers can experience positive transformation and growth, they may never feel "the same." The key point here is that in normal grief one regains a sense of meaning and purpose. In complicated grief, the person cannot find any way to accept the loss and make sense of it. The acute distress continues, without relief. The core features of complicated grief include intrusive thoughts related to the deceased, intense pain of separation distress, and distressingly strong yearnings for the deceased. Because normal grief is a natural process, it generally does not require professional help. On the other hand, in complicated grief professional intervention is needed. When acute grief is not progressively integrated into a new paradigm, the griever may continue to experience severe yearning, separation distress, and cognitive distortions about the death even several years after the event[71–73] (see Chapter 5 for assessment considerations).

Different frameworks have been developed to describe complicated grief, based on researchers' conceptualization of the phenomenon and the research focus. Some of the terms that have also been used in the past are abnormal grief, complicated mourning, chronic grief, and traumatic grief. It has been argued that *complicated mourning* would be a more appropriate term, because it highlights that it is not the experience of grief that is pathological, but mourning, that is, the intrapsychic process by which individuals are able to integrate the loss into a new and meaningful life framework.[23]

Although some symptoms of complicated grief overlap with symptoms of major depression and posttraumatic stress disorder, the core features of complicated grief are distinct from the psychiatric disorders included in *DSM-IV* as demonstrated by the work of Horowitz, Prigerson, and Shear.[74–76] As a result, complicated grief was proposed as a newly recognized disorder and diagnostic entity different from major depression and anxiety.

Even though the grief and bereavement field is evolving quickly, the available studies have recruited mostly white bereaved women, limiting the generalizability of the results to other populations of bereaved, such as men, minorities, children, and older grievers. Based on these limitations, recent work in the areas has questioned the construct validity of complicated grief as compared to other bereavement outcomes.[77] The suggestion of including complicated grief as a psychiatric disorder in *The Diagnostic and Statistical Manual of Mental Disorders*, fifth edition (*DSM-5*) has generated significant controversy. The recent release of the *DSM-5* has suspended the debate: complicated grief has not been included as a separate diagnostic category, but it is proposed as an adjustment reaction related to bereavement. Nonetheless, the existence of complicated grief is recognized by the majority of researchers, clinicians, and scholars in the field.

Complicated grief has been associated with increased risk for hypertension, cardiac events, disability, reduced quality of life, and suicidal ideation and behaviors.[62,63,78] Complicated grief is also associated with lower self-concept clarity[65] and associated with grievers' diminished ability to formulate personal goals focused on social, recreational, and occupational activities.[66] Additionally, complicated grief negatively affects grievers' ability to imagine a positive future not focused on loss.[67] Studies have suggested that complicated grief affects autobiographic and self-defining memories.[68,69] Individuals with complicated grief report memories related to the deceased as more defining of their sense of identity. Additionally, they appear to find less benefit from recalling memories of the loved one, when compared to a group of non-complicated grievers. There is also indication that complicated grief affects physiological correlates, such as cortisol levels, which did not show normal diurnal variation during the day in a group of 12 women with complicated grief, compared to a control group.[70]

The discussion in the complicated grief literature has focused primarily on bereaved family members and other caregivers after the death of someone close. As a result, it may be easy to forget that patients with advanced illness may also be experiencing complicated grief, with present losses compounding unprocessed losses in the past.

References

1. Zisook S, Devaul RA, Click MA, Jr. Measuring symptoms of grief and bereavement. *Am J Psychiatry* 1982;139(12):1590–3.

2. Clieren M. *Bereavement and Adaptation: A Comparative Study of the Aftermath of Death*. Washington, DC: Hemisphere Publishing; 1993.

3. Raphael B, Dobson M. Bereavement. In: Harvey JH, Miller ED, eds. *Loss and Trauma*. Philadelphia, PA: Brunner Routledge; 2000: 45–61.

4. Sprang G, McNeil J. *The Many Faces of Bereavement: The Nature and Treatment of Natural, Traumatic, and Stigmatized Grief*. New York: Brunner/Mazel; 1995.

5. Cottington EM, Matthews KA, Talbott E, et al. Environmental events preceding sudden deaths in women. *Psychosomatic Med* 1980;42:567–74.

6. Lindstrom TC. Immunity and health after bereavement in relation to coping. *Scand J Psychol* 1997;38:253–9.

7. Manor O, Eisenbach Z. Mortality after spousal loss: are there socio-demographic differences? *SocSci Med* 2003;56(2):405–13.

8. Hart CL, Hole DJ, Lawlor DA, et al. Effect of conjugal bereavement on mortality of the bereaved spouse in participants of the Renfrew/Paisley Study. *J Epidemiol Community Health* 2007;61(5):455–60.

9. Jones DR, Goldblatt PO. Causes of death in widowers and spouses. *J Biosocial Sci* 1987;19:107–21.

10. Ajdacic-Gross V, Ring M, Gadola E, et al. Suicide after bereavement: an overlooked problem. *Psychological Med* 2008;38(5):673–6.

11. Erlangsen A, Jeune B, Bille-Brahe U, et al. Loss of partner and suicide risks among oldest old: a population-based register study. *Age Ageing* 2004;33(4): 378–83.

12. Hansen NB, Vaughan EL, Cavanaugh CE, Connell CM, Sikkema KJ. Health-related quality of life in bereaved HIV-positive adults: relationships between HIV symptoms, grief, social support, and Axis II indication. *Health Psychol* 2009;28(2):249–57.

13. Breitbart W, Gibson C, Tremblay A. The delirium experience: delirium recall and delirium-related distress in hospitalized patients with cancer, their spouses/ caregivers, and their nurses. *Psychosomatics* 2002;43(3):183–94.

14. Breitbart W, Alici Y. Agitation and delirium at the end of life: "We could not manage him." *JAMA* 2008;300(24):2898–910.

15. Irwin M, Daniels M, Weiner H. Immune and neuro-endocrine changes after bereavement. *Psychiatric Clin North Am* 1987;10:449–65.

16. Schleifer S, Keller M, Camerino J, et al. Suppression of lymphocytes stimulation following bereavement. *JAMA* 1983;250:374–7.

17. Hensley PL, Clayton PJ. Bereavement: signs, symptoms, and course. *Psychiatr Ann* 2008;38:649–54.

18. O'Connor MF, Irwin MR, Wellish DK. When grief heats up: pro-inflammatory cytokines predict regional brain activation. *Neuroimage* 2009;47(3):891–6.

19. Walsh K, King M, Jones L, et al. Spiritual beliefs may affect outcome of bereavement: prospective study. *BMJ* 2002;324:1551.

20. King M, Speck P, Thomas A. The effect of spiritual beliefs on outcome from illness. *Soc Sci Med* 1999;48:1291–9.

21. Rando TA. *Grief, Dying, and Death: Clinical Interventions for Caregivers.* Champaign, IL: Research Press, 1984.

22. Worden JW. *Grief Counseling and Grief Therapy: A Handbook for the Mental Health Professional.* 4th ed. New York: Springer; 2009.

23. Rando TA. *Treatment of Complicated Mourning.* Champaign, IL: Research Press; 1993.

24. Lindemann E. The symptomatology and management of acute grief. *Am J Psychiatry* 1944;101:141–8.

25. Fulton G, Madden C, Minichiello V. The social construction of anticipatory grief. *Soc Sci Med* 1996;43(9):1349–58.

26. Evans AJ. Anticipatory grief: a theoretical challenge. *Palliat Med* 1994;8(2):159–65.

27. Sweeting HN, Gilhooly ML. Anticipatory grief: a review. *Soc Sci Med* 1990;30(10):1073–80.

28. Reynolds L, Botha D. Anticipatory grief: its nature, impact, and reasons for contradictory findings. *Couns, Psychother Health* 2006;2(2):15–26.

29. Cheng JO, Lo RS, Chan FM, Kwan BH, Woo J. An exploration of anticipatory grief in advanced cancer patients. *Psychooncology* 2010;19(7):693–700.

30. Holley CK, Mast BT. The impact of anticipatory grief on caregiver burden in dementia caregivers. *Gerontologist* 2009;49(3):388–96.

31. Gilliland G, Fleming S. A comparison of spousal anticipatory grief and conventional grief. *Death Studies* 1998;22(6):541–69.

32. Duke S. An exploration of anticipatory grief: the lived experience of people during their spouses' terminal illness and in bereavement. *J Adv Nurs* 1998;28(4):829–39.

33. Chapman KJ, Pepler C. Coping, hope, and anticipatory grief in family members in palliative home care. *Cancer Nurs* 1998;21(4):226–34.

34. Coombs MA. The mourning before: can anticipatory grief theory inform family care in adult intensive care? *Int J Palliat Nurs* 16(12):580–584.

35. Wong MS, Chan SW. The experiences of Chinese family members of terminally ill patients-a qualitative study. *J Clin Nurs* 2007;16(12):2357–64.

36. Mystakidou K, Parpa E, Tsilika E, et al. Preparatory grief, psychological distress and hopelessness in advanced cancer patients. *Eur J Cancer Care (Engl)* 2008;17(2):145–51.

37. Mystakidou K, Tsilika E, Parpa E, et al. Illness-related hopelessness in advanced cancer: influence of anxiety, depression, and preparatory grief. *Arch Psychiatr Nurs* 2009;23(2):138–47.

38. Garand L, Lingler H, et al. (2011). Anticipatory grief in new family caregivers of persons with mild cognitive impairment and dementia. *Alzheimer Dis Assoc Disord*, Sept. 22, 2011.

39. Holley CK, Mast BT. The impact of anticipatory grief on caregiver burden in dementia caregivers. *Gerontologist* 2009;49(3):338–396.

40. Frank JB. Evidence for grief as the major barrier faced by Alzheimer caregiver: a qualitative analysis. *Am J Alzheimer Dis Other Demen* 2007;22(6):516–27.

41. Johansson AK, Grimby. Anticipatory grief among close relatives of patients at hospice and palliative wards. *Am J Hosp Palliat Care*, May 19, 2011.

42. Pusa S, Persson C, et al. Significant others' lived experiences following a lung cancer trajectory: from diagnosis through and after the death of a family member. *Eur J Oncol Nurs* 2012;16(1):34–41.

43. Anngela-cole L, Busch L. Stress and grief among family caregivers of older adults with cancer: a multicultural comparison from Hawaii. *J Soc Work End Life Palliat Care* 2011;7(4):318–37.

44. Peteet JR, Maytal G, et al. Unimaginable loss: contingent suicidal ideation in family members of oncology patients. *Psychosomatics* 2010;51(2):166–70.

45. Lobb EA, Clayton JM, Price MA. Suffering, loss and grief in palliative care. *Aust Fam Physician* 2006;35(10):772–5.

46. Periyakoil VS, Hallenbeck J. Identifying and managing preparatory grief and depression at the end of life. *Am Fam Physician* 2002;65(5):883–90.

47. Tsilika E, Mystakidou K, Parpa E, Galanos A, Sakkas P, Vlahos L. The influence of cancer impact on patients' preparatory grief. *Psychol Health* 2009;24(2):135–48.

48. Mystakidou K, Tsilika E, Parpa E, et al. Demographic and clinical predictors of preparatory grief in a sample of advanced cancer patients. *Psychooncology* 2006;15(9):828–33.

49. Kubler-Ross, E. *On death and dying*. New York: Macmillan, 1969.

50. Hottensen D. Anticipatory grief in patients with cancer. *Clin J Oncol Nurs* 2010;14(1):106–7.

51. Glaser BG, Strauss AL. *Awareness of Dying*. Chicago: Aldine Transactions, 1965.

52. Mystakidou K, Tsilika E, Parpa E, Galanos A, Vlahos L. Screening for preparatory grief in advanced cancer patients. *Cancer Nurs* 2008;31(4):326–32.

53. Marwit SJ, Meuser TM. Development and initial validation of an inventory to assess grief in caregivers of persons with Alzheimer's disease. *Gerontologist* 2002;42(6):751–65.

54. Buckley T, Sunari D, Marshall A, et al. Physiological correlates of bereavement and the impact of bereavement interventions. *Dialogues Clin Neurosci* 2012;14:129–39.

55. Buckley T, McKinley S, Tofler G, Bartrop R. Cardiovascular risk in early bereavement: a literature review and proposed mechanisms. *Int J Nurs Stud* 2010;47(2):229–38.

56. Khanfer R, Lord JM, Phillips AC. Neutrophil function and cortisol: DHEAS ratio in bereaved older adults. *Brain Behav Immun* 2011;25(6):1182–6.

57. Hart C, Hole D, Lawlor D, et al. Effect of conjugal bereavement on mortality of the bereaved spouse in participants of the Renfrew/Paisley Study. *J Epidemiol Community Health* 2007;61:455–60.

58. Shear MK, Skritskaya NA. Bereavement and anxiety. *Curr Psychiatry Rep* 2012;14(3):169–75.

59. Shear MK. Getting straight about grief. *Dep Anx* 2012;29(6):46–4.

60. Byrne GJ, Raphael B. The psychological symptoms of conjugal bereavement in elderly men over the first 13 months. *Int Geriatr Psychiatry* 1997;12(2):241–51.

61. Miller MD. Complicated grief in late life. *Dialogues Clin Neurosci* 2012;14:195–202.

62. Boelen PA, Prigerson HG. The influence of prolonged grief disorder, depression and anxiety on quality of life among bereaved adults. *Eur Arch Psychiatry Clin Neurosci* 2007;257:444–52.

63. Newson RS, Boelen PA, Hek K, et al. The prevalence and characteristics of complicated grief in older adults. *J Affect Disord* 2011;132(1–2):231–8.

64. MacKenzie M. Preparatory grief in frail elderly individuals. *Annals of Long Term Care* 2011;19(1):22–26.

65. Boelen PA, Keijsers L, van den Hout MA. The role of self-concept clarity in prolonged grief disorder. *J Nerv Ment Dis* 2012;200(1):56–62.

66. Boelen, PA. Personal goals and prolonged grief disorder symptoms. *Clin Psychol Psychother* 2011;18(6):439–44.

67. Maccallum F, Bryant RA. Imagining the future in complicated grief. *Depress Anxiety* 2011;28(8):658–65.

68. Maccallum F, Bryant RA. Self-defining memories in complicated grief. *Behav Res* 2008;46(12):1311–15.

69. Maccallum F, Bryant RA. Impaired autobiographical memory in complicated grief. *Behav Res Ther* 2010;48(4):328–34.

70. O'Connor MF, Wellisch DK, Stanton AL, Olmstead R, Irwin MR. Diurnal cortisol in complicated and non-complicated grief: slope differences across the day. *Psychoneuroendocrinology* 2012;37(5):725–8.

71. Zisook S, Simon NM, Reynolds CF, et al. Bereavement, complicated grief, and DSM, part 2:complicated grief. *J Clin Psychiatr* 2010;71:1097–8.

72. Shear K, Shair H. Attachment, loss, and complicated grief. *Dev Psychobiol* 2005;47(3):253–67.

73. Monk TH, Houck PR, Shear MK. The daily life of complicated grief patients – what gets missed, what gets added? *Death Studies* 2006;30(1):77–85.

74. Horowitz MJ, Siegel B, Holen A, Bonanno GA, et al. Diagnostic criteria for complicated grief disorder. *Am J Psychiatry* 1997;154(7):904–10.

75. Forstmeier S, Maercker A. Comparison of two diagnostic systems for complicated grief. *J Affect Disord* 2007;99(1–3):203–11.

76. Shear KM, Simon N, Wall M, Zisook S, Neimeyer R, et al. Complicated grief and related bereavement issues for the DSM-5. *Depress Anx* 2011;28:103–17.

77. Shah SN, Meeks S. Late-life bereavement and complicated grief: a proposed comprehensive framework. *Aging Ment Health* 2012;16(1):39–56.

78. Szanto K, Shear MK, Houck PR, et al. indirect self-destructive behavior and overt suicidality in patients with complicated grief. *J Clin Psychiatry* 2006;67(2)233–9.

Clinical and Professional Considerations

Chapter 5

Assessment Considerations

Focus Points

- Grief and bereavement assessment should begin at the first contact between the palliative care or hospice team and the patient and family.
- The assessment process need not be overly formal or overly structured, but it can become a therapeutic intervention for the patient and family when conducted with cultural sensitivity, cultural humility, and cultural competence.
- A thorough assessment may require more than one visit with the patient and the family and may be the result of various contributions from various members of the interdisciplinary team. Whenever possible, appropriate, and clinically indicated, patients and families should also be evaluated separately.
- Anticipatory grief in family caregivers should be regularly monitored and supported by the team. Risk factors and protective factors should be also be identified and regularly monitored.
- Preparatory (anticipatory) grief in patients is a natural and non-pathological process that should be validated and supported with adequate psychosocial and spiritual interventions. It generally does not warrant pharmacological intervention. While they are different, preparatory grief and depression may be comorbid.
- Depression in patients with advanced illness should be diagnosed focusing primarily on psychological symptoms, especially anhedonia (loss of pleasure), hopelessness, sense of worthlessness, and persistent low mood. Depending on the patient's prognosis and overall condition, it must be actively treated with psychotherapy, medication, or a combination of both.
- Complicated grief is a disabling condition caused by acute grief for the death of a close person that is not integrated into the griever's psyche. It can affect both patients with advanced illness and caregivers and it warrants evaluation and intervention by a mental health professional.
- Bereavement-related depression can be triggered by the stress of losing someone close. It indicates a pathological process that must be recognized and actively treated. According to the new edition of the Diagnostic and Statistic Manual of Mental Disorders (DSM-5), grievers who meet full criteria can be diagnosed with Major Depression, even though they may still be in the process of acute grief. Clinicians need to develop expertise in recognizing the difference between normal grief and depression; this is crucial to avoid

pathologizing a normal grieving process or overdiagnosing depression during acute grief.

Grief and bereavement assessment of patients with advanced illness and their family caregivers is a necessary and important task for palliative care clinicians. The diagnostic information obtained can be used to correctly identify grief reactions in patients and caregivers and to monitor "symptom" severity. A meaningful assessment allows clinicians should not only to recognize the extent and nature of patients and caregivers' grief reactions, but also to understand the interaction with cultural, spiritual, and psychosocial aspects, essential for the development of a treatment plan.[1]

The terms *screening* and *assessment* are often used interchangeably, but the basic differences are worth reviewing.

Screening is a relatively quick but nonetheless specific process that allows the clinician to identify areas of concern. The extent of the level of concern determines the initial plan and the need for in-depth exploration by a clinical assessment. In essence, grief and bereavement screening identifies area of concerns and "red flags" that may indicate a higher risk level and should be explored by assessment. Clinical assessment is a longer, in-depth, and ongoing process that allows clinicians to define the nature of the problem more precisely and to develop diagnostic conclusions and an appropriate treatment plan.[2]

Ideally, all members of the interdisciplinary palliative care team will be able to perform a relatively quick screening during the initial contact with patients and caregivers, including grief-specific questions. For example, it is useful to ask the following:

- Is any other family member currently ill?
- Has the family sustained a loss from death in the previous 2 years?
- Can the family rely on adequate social support?
- Are there any other stressors/losses that may trigger grief reactions, even if not directly related to the illness? For example, if a patient's spouse becomes unemployed, there may be not only serious financial repercussions but also grief reactions elicited by loss of stability, loss of status, and loss of a sense of personal identity. Similarly, stressors affecting patients' close family members will inevitably result in additional grief and sadness for the entire family. The impact of these situations on patients and families may appear obvious, but it should not be underestimated, even if not directly connected to the illness. Clinicians will not know unless they gently explore.

One patient commented feeling devastated when she was told that her breast cancer had spread to her bones and lungs, but she felt she could handle it. A few months later her only daughter had a miscarriage and a hysterectomy due to the complications. At every visit the patient told the palliative care team that her grief and worry were focused on her daughter and that she would not and could not discuss her physical pain because it was "nothing" compared to what she was feeling as a mother and a grandmother. She felt her daughter's pregnancy represented her only opportunity to become a grandmother, and now it had vanished. She became withdrawn and avoidant toward the family. The psychosocial/psychological treatment plan in this case focused on helping the patient process the grief for the miscarriage and the grief for the loss of her anticipated role. Only after the patient developed a way of considering the loss that was meaningful to her was she able to refocus on her illness and allow herself to have her pain treated, which in turn allowed her to continue to engage fully with her family until her death, 5 months later. Using this case as an example, a brief screening may allow palliative care clinicians to know that the patient's daughter suffered a miscarriage and a hysterectomy. However, only the clinical interview allows for the development of a more complete understanding of the meaning and the extent of the loss for the patient and the rest of the family. Thus, it is not only important to identify possible sources of grief; it is also important to understand the meaning and manifestations of the stressor, including how it may affect the patient's current status and treatment.

Any member of the interdisciplinary palliative care team can ask grief-related questions, but coordination and appropriate information sharing with the team are especially important. First, it is not uncommon for patients to disclose different parts of their loss history or current grief reactions with different clinicians. Therefore, team members should develop an integrated and consistent clinical understanding of the patient and caregivers based on all the available information obtained by different clinicians at different times. Apparent inconsistencies in the description of the family story should be approached with caution and sensitivity, remembering that it is common for patients to emphasize different parts of their experience, at different times, with different people. Secondly, after initial screening information is obtained, it is helpful to discuss whether the family needs a primary psychosocial clinician involved in continuing to provide assessment, monitoring, and interventions. The goal is not to promote territoriality or prevent other clinicians from exploring grief reactions in their work. However, it is also important that patients and families do not feel burdened by different clinicians repeatedly asking the same questions. Therefore, knowledge of the family style is crucial. Some patients and families clearly welcome support from every clinician on the team and will gladly volunteer information, benefiting from a variety of different interventions. Other patients and caregivers may be significantly more private and selective in their disclosure and willingness to discuss psychosocial or psychological concerns and may express frustration if several clinicians approach them. Clinicians often develop intuitions about whether patients and families prefer exploring and processing their grief with different clinicians, or whether they prefer confidential conversations with only one. However, clinical intuitions should always be thoroughly explored during the clinical interview and therefore confirmed or disconfirmed. In this way, clinicians will avoid making assumptions about family preferences, which may be more reflective of clinicians' biases than actual assessment of needs.[3]

The Clinical Interview as Therapeutic Intervention

To minimize burden, it may be useful to include exploration of grief reactions as part of the initial psychosocial interview. The nature of the settings, the patient's ability and willingness to engage in the interview process, and the presence of family members participating in the interview will determine the length of the meeting.

A thorough assessment with palliative care patients may require more than one meeting, but it should not be burdensome for the patient. The purpose of the assessment is obtaining information to develop a plan to help the patient. However, patients and caregivers should feel that they are being given "something back" at the time of assessment. This approach will not only be focused on obtaining adequate information and assessing risk level but also on providing interventions that may be immediately beneficial and relieve suffering.

For example, supportive education about grief reactions (see Chapter 6), validation of the grief experience, and normalization of grief phenomenology can be provided during the interview, allowing clinicians to provide a sort of "therapeutic assessment." Furthermore, palliative care patients and family caregivers are often acutely aware of how time is spent, especially when there is awareness of a limited prognosis. Provision of appropriate grief-related interventions during assessment honors and maximizes that precious time.

Table 5.1 presents a template for assessment of grief and bereavement. It indicates areas that could be explored during the interview. It can be used to explore grief reactions both in patients and family caregivers. Clinicians can

---

Table 5.1 Grief and Bereavement Interview

1. Explore the circumstances of initial diagnosis and course of treatment. How did the patient and the family process the losses and challenges? If the patient does not wish to discuss, this information can be obtained from family caregivers, or clinicians who have cared for the patient in the past.

2. Explore the nature of previous transitions of care and associated grief reactions at each stage. The goal is not to re-traumatize the patient and the family, but to obtain information about personal and family grieving styles. For example, do patients and caregivers have similar grieving styles? Is there conflict in the family regarding how emotions, including grief, are expressed?

3. Does the patient have a spiritual or religious orientation? If yes, is it supporting the patient and/or caregivers *at this time*? If yes, how? If the answer is no, is the patient grieving loss of faith or loss of spiritual resources? Do patients and family members share a connection to spiritual resources? Or, is spirituality/religion a possible source of conflict? Is the patient/family experiencing spiritual distress that warrants referral to a spiritual care professional?

4. What has been the relationship to the prior treating team? Does the treating physician/oncologist maintain contact with the patient? Does the patient wish to be visited by his or her oncologist, even if disease-modifying treatment has been stopped? Does the patient feel "abandoned" if the oncologist does not visit?

Table 5.1 Continued

5. What is the predominant communication style in the family. How is conflict handled? Do family members openly discuss emotions? Are decisions made cooperatively or by one specific family member? How has the illness modified the communication style? Are there grief reactions associated with these changes?

6. Level of death awareness in the family system: open, closed, suspected awareness, mutual pretense. Is the illness openly discussed in the family? Is indirect language used to refer to the illness? Does the level of shared awareness seem to be supportive of the patient and the family or is it causing increased distress?

7. Is anyone experiencing *disenfranchised grief*? For example, are there estranged family members or friends, or former spouses, who may still feel connected to the patient but are not part of the close circle of support? Is this issue a source of suffering for the patient and the family?

8. Explore the presence of physical and symbolic losses in the past two years NOT related to the illness: assess patient, family, community (loss of job, death of other family members, difficulties related to immigration issues, natural disasters in home country for immigrants, etc.)

9. Is anyone experiencing complicated grief (aka *prolonged grief*), bereavement-related depression, or anxiety disorders? Remember to assess the patient, as well as the caregivers

10. *Patient assessment*: recognize preparatory grief vs. depression. Recognize complicated grief.

11. *Caregiver assessment*: recognize anticipatory grief vs. depression vs. grieving style not acknowledged or addressed vs. difficult family dynamics, especially ambivalence

12. *Current Risk factors for patient and family caregivers*: previous history of mental health difficulties, especially depression; ambivalent relationship with patient and/or caregivers, history of domestic violence, abuse, addiction, health problems, psychosocial, cultural aspects, financial stressors. Identify placement/discharge challenges that may generate severe grief reactions (e.g. patient wants to return home, but the caregiver is unwilling or unable to continue providing continual care. Or, a patient previously living alone is not longer able to return home and will need to move to a facility.

13. *Protective factors for patients and family caregivers*: social support, individual characteristics and adaptive defense mechanisms (resilience, humor, etc.), supportive spiritual/religious beliefs, and/or community.

14. Is a referral indicated? *For Patients* → Specialist level palliative care: social work and psychology? Psychiatric consultation? Palliative care attending as prescriber if psychotropic medication is needed? Need for coordination with primary team.

For Caregivers → Referrals to outpatient psychiatry and/or psychology. Consider referrals to primary care physicians for further evaluation and treatment.

Assess for Presence of vulnerable caregivers, i.e., grandparents.

Children in the family → What is the developmental stage? How much information has been given/should be given to the child? Monitor acting out in school; recognize symptoms of depression/anxiety. Does the family need education about developmentally appropriate strategies to support grieving children?

Adapted and modified from Strada EA. The Helping Professional's Guide to End of Life Care. Oakland, CA: New Harbinger, 2013 modify it according to the nature of their setting and the patient's situation. The therapeutic stance adopted by the clinician is key here. As mentioned previously, assessing a patient for grief reactions involves more than following a template or a checklist. Each point represents a possible area for exploration. Each moment of exploration requires establishing an empathic and emotionally "safe" environment.

In the last decade several standardized measures have been developed and are routinely used in research. While they can be very helpful to identify pathological grief reactions, they cannot replace an in-depth clinical interview. Structured tools can help clinicians obtain a quick picture of areas of concerns and symptoms, and even allow formulation of *DSM*-based diagnoses; however, only the clinical interview conducted with cultural sensitivity, empathy, and compassion can allow the full understanding of the meaning and depth of symptoms and concerns, thus facilitating development and implementation of individualized treatment plans. Additionally, despite the recent growth of bereavement research and the development of structured assessment tools in the palliative care setting, there is currently no clear gold standard. A recent review of available bereavement measurable tools has pointed out the theoretical and statistical weaknesses that make implementation challenging.[4]

Assessment of Anticipatory Grief in Family Caregivers

The level of distress experienced by family caregivers is well-documented;[5–8] it may be argued that the caregiving for a family member with advanced illness represents a risk factor in itself. Anticipatory grief in family caregivers has been associated with significant emotional distress, cognitive dysfunction, irritability, social isolation, and loneliness.[9–11,15] Therefore, to implement an adequate plan it is important that the team identifies additional risk factors that may be present, and sources of support and protective factors that may assist the caregiver.

A history of difficult relationship with a high level of ambivalence between the patient and the family caregiver can represent a risk factor for high levels of anticipatory grief. Clinicians must remember, however, that anticipatory grief in family caregivers is not necessarily only related to the loss that will occur with the death of the loved one. Rather, it is a process of mourning all the concrete and symbolic losses that have occurred since diagnosis and the beginning of the journey through illness and transitions of care.[12] Sudden and apparently maladaptive changes in the caregiver's behavior, either toward the patient or the treating team (Table 5.2), may be indicative of increasing and unmanageable distress. Caregivers who exhibit severe and unmanageable levels of anticipatory grief should become a priority for the palliative care team and receive frequent and ongoing assessment, monitoring, and interventions. Caregivers presenting with moderate to severe symptoms of depression and/or anxiety, or symptoms of other psychiatric disorders should be assessed by team members with specialized mental health training. Possible interventions may include referrals

Table 5.2 Caregivers' Behaviors That May Raise Concern

- Caregiver exhibits severe self-neglect (refuses to eat regularly, stops taking prescribed medication).

- Caregiver exhibits sudden change in behavior toward patient (from close involvement to overt avoidance or detachment).

- Caregiver begins talking about the patient using the past tense, as though the death has already occurred. This behavior may be concurrent with severe grief symptoms, as expected in early phases of bereavement.

- As the patient's physical decline continues, caregiver begins expressing overt and increasing anger, repulsion, and disgust about physical changes in the patient's body.

- Caregiver demonstrates continuous and persistent inability/refusal to process/ integrate information about the patient's prognosis; may start demanding that medical team provide interventions/treatments considered medically contraindicated and likely to cause undue pain/suffering for the patient.

to primary care physicians, contacting other family members to ensure safety, grief counseling, or grief therapy (see Chapter 6) provided during their visits at the hospital.

Risk assessment always needs to be determined when caregivers express suicidal ideation, even if it is passive. The following should be evaluated:

- Is the caregiver aware of the patient's prognosis? Does the caregiver have reasonable expectations about the patient's prognosis? Will the caregiver be surprised by the patient's death?

- Is the caregiver able to imagine a life after the patient's death?

- Is the caregiver making suicidal comments, even in passing, such as "I will not be able to go on after he/she dies"; I can't survive his/her death"; or "Nothing is going to help me after he/she dies"? If these or similar comments are made, it is appropriate to perform a complete suicidal assessment to determine risk.

- Is the caregiver expressing active suicidal ideation? Are the three components of suicidal ideation present (i.e., intent, plan, means)? If the caregiver is actively suicidal, strategies must be put into place to maintain safety (e.g., alerting family members, psychiatric evaluation). Clinicians should not automatically assume that suicidal ideation is simply an expression of distress and the caregiver will not act on it.

Assessment of Preparatory (Anticipatory) Grief in Patients with Advanced Illness

Emotional distress in patients with advanced illness has commonly been assessed by using general measures of psychiatric disorders, such as measures of depression and anxiety. However, whilst preparatory grief may cause emotional distress for the patient, it does not represent a pathological process. Preparatory grief can be conceptualized as somewhat similar to normal grief after the death of a loved one; it can feel intensely painful, but it generally represents a normal developmental process involved in adjustment to a significant loss. As mentioned previously (see Chapter 4), patients with advanced illness and patients who are approaching death are often engaged in grieving several losses, including adjusting to the idea of their own life ending soon.[13,14] Their grieving process should be recognized and supported, while monitoring for the development of disorders, such as major depression, which may develop if the pain of preparatory grief becomes unmanageable. It ensues that development of measures designed to specifically assess grief reactions in patients with advanced illness and differentiate them from disorders such as depression is an important emerging area in the literature and especially clinically relevant for this population.

In an effort to address this need, Mystakidou et al.[16–19] developed the Preparatory Grief in Advanced Cancer Patients Scale (PGAC), which is a 31-item self-report measure designed to measure levels of preparatory grief in patients with advanced cancer. Because preparatory grief is a normal and adaptive process, the purpose of this measure is not to distinguish between normal and "pathological preparatory grief." Rather, it is intended to recognize levels of grief in several areas that have been described as relevant to patients with advanced cancer.[16] On the other hand, while normal, preparatory grief may increase to such intensity to become unmanageable for the patient. Thus, it has been suggested that high levels of preparatory grief could become a risk factor for increased distress.[16] The PGAC contains 7 subscales that represent the psychological, interpersonal, and sociocultural aspects of preparatory grief, addressing the following domains: (1) self-consciousness, (2) disease adjustment, (3) sadness, (4) anger, (5) religious comfort, (6) somatic symptoms, and (7) perceived social support. Patients are asked to rank their level of agreement with the items on a 4-point Likert scale. Because the measure is not intended to assess pathology, the authors do not recommend a specific cutoff. However, it is suggested that patients who endorse high levels of preparatory grief, as indicated by high levels of distress in each of the subscales, should receive further evaluation, in the form of a clinical interview to explore in depth the sources of distress and provide adequate psychosocial and spiritual support.

Because preparatory grief is a natural developmental process, it needs to be recognized as such, supported, and distinguished from other entities with similar symptoms, such as depression. This is not always easy because, as mentioned previously, patients with advanced illness who are experiencing preparatory grief may present very distressed. Low mood, sadness, crying, social withdrawal, and anxiety can be present in preparatory grief as well as in depression. Correct recognition of the patient's experience is crucial, because diagnosis drives treatment.[20–22,25,27–29]

Differentiating Preparatory Grief from Depression in Patients

While preparatory grief can elicit intense negative affect, it is different from major depression. In the most severe cases preparatory grief and depression can be comorbid, and treatment may include a combination of medication and therapy. However, whenever possible, it is important to differentiate between the two, because patients in preparatory grief need to be adequately supported by psychotherapy interventions that specifically address grief-related existential and spiritual distress.

As a general guideline, patients who are experiencing major depression or bereavement-related depression experience no fluctuation in mood and report anhedonia as a core element of their experience. Patients who are grieving may appear depressed, but they generally retain the ability to experience positive emotions, even though their mood, affect, and ability to engage fluctuate. Patients who are grieving may experience guilt related to past actions or activities; however, this is generally related to specific events, and not pervasive. On the other hand, patients who are depressed may experience pervasive feelings or worthlessness and irrational guilt that appear unrelated to the patient's situation. One patient with advanced illness and major depression described himself in the following terms " I am just a pathetic human being and I want to end it. No reason; I am just pathetic and a waste" (Table 5.3).

The intensity of distress in preparatory grief can develop into a major depressive episode, especially in patients at high risk for depression. Therefore,

Table 5.3 Differentiating Preparatory Grief from Depression in Palliative Care Patients

Preparatory Grief	Depression
• Mood fluctuates. There may be moments of profound distress, crying, and anxiety, followed by positive affect.	• The patient feels sad or low most of the time, tearful. Affect appears generally flat.
• Self-esteem is generally intact. The patient may experience feelings of guilt related to life choices he/she thinks are related to current situation (e.g. alcohol or drug abuse, cigarette smoking). However, guilt is not irrational and is not pervasive.	• Constant feelings of worthlessness and guilt. These feelings are pervasive and not usually connected to identifiable causes or to the illness.
• The patient is able to enjoy seeing and interacting with friends and family. Still, there may be fluctuation in the patient's ability and desire to engage with others.	• The patient withdraws from friends and family; less talkative. However, this withdrawal/disengagement may be natural and adaptive in patients who are very close to dying.
• The patient is able to experience pleasure in various activities that are meaningful.	• Anhedonia. The patient experiences a loss of interest in activities that were previously considered meaningful. There is a sense that nothing can be done to improve the patient's mood, even temporarily
• The patient is able to look forward to special occasions, e.g. grandchildren's birthdays, a visit from a relative living out of state. In moments of profound distress patients may experience suicidal ideation and verbalize a wish to die. However this is mostly passive and temporary.	• Frequent thoughts of early death, or suicide. May frequently ask physicians to hasten death. Suicidality assessment may be needed.

identifying risk factors for depression should be a priority of the palliative care team and a major focus of the initial assessment. Unrecognized and untreated major depression creates significant suffering for patients and caregivers and is associated with suicidal ideation and increased requests for hastened death in terminal patients.[23,24]

The research literature provides inconsistent data about the prevalence of depression in patients with advanced illness. It has been estimated that rates of major depression in patients who are dying can vary from 22% to 75%.[28] These differences may depend on a number of factors, including cultural variables and differences in the settings where the studies were conducted. One of the most relevant methodological factors affecting the discrepancy in reported prevalence is the different threshold for diagnosing depression in the various studies. Studies that utilize a low threshold will likely include those with minor depression and adjustment disorders, while studies utilizing more stringent criteria and higher threshold will include only the more severe cases of depression. As a result, the reported prevalence can vary substantially, demonstrating that diagnosing major depression in patients with advanced illness and their loved ones can be challenging.

While the term *depression* is sometimes used to indicate a variety of situations where the patient feels low, or sad, a diagnosis of major depression means *DSM* defining criteria are met. However, it is well known that many of the somatic symptoms of depression, such as fatigue, disturbances in the sleep cycle, loss of energy, and weight loss are common in patients with advanced illness. Thus, it has been suggested that clinicians focus on patients' psychological symptoms and not on somatic symptoms in the assessment process.[27] Utilizing the substitutive approach suggested by Endicott can assist palliative clinicians.[26] According to the substitutive method, weight loss or gain should be substituted with depressed appearance; insomnia or hypersomnia with social withdrawal or decreased talkativeness; psychomotor agitation or retardation with brooding, self-pity, or pessimism; and diminished ability to concentrate or indecisiveness with lack of reactivity and inability to be cheered up. Table 5.4 presents the *DSM-IV* criteria for major depression and Endicott's substitutive criteria.

Because of their focus on somatic symptoms, the majority of self-report screening tools may not be appropriate for use with palliative care patients. Additionally, as patients' illness progresses and their overall level of function declines, they may have difficulty reading the questions and completing the tools. Among the screening tools utilized in palliative care research, the Hospital Anxiety and Depression Scale (HADS) excludes most of the somatic complaints associated with depression, focusing on emotional complaints, and has been widely used in patients with advanced illness.[30]

Chochinov and colleagues studied a simple screening option and found that simply asking patients directly the question "Are you depressed?" was effective in screening for patients who, on subsequent assessment, met criteria for major depression.[31] As a result of this study, the American Society of Internal Medicine has endorsed the inclusion of this depression screening question in the care of patients with advanced illness. Notwithstanding the value of self-administered and

Table 5.4 Symptoms of Major Depression According to the *DSM* and Endicott's Criteria

DSM-IV-TR	Endicott
Depressed mood most of the day OR markedly diminished interest or pleasure in all, or almost all, activities most of the day	
Weight loss or gain	Depressed appearance
Insomnia or hypersomnia	Social withdrawal or decreased talkativeness
Psychomotor agitation or retardation	
Fatigue or loss of energy	Brooding, self-pity, or pessimism
Diminished ability to concentrate, or indecisiveness	Lack of reactivity; cannot be cheered up
Recurrent thoughts of death, suicidal ideation or planning, or a suicide attempt	

clinician screening tools, the clinical interview is the standard for diagnosing major depression and should be considered in all cases where questions remain.

Periyakoil et al.[32] developed a the Terminally Ill Grief or Depression Scale to help differentiate grief from depression in patients with advanced illness. Their measure is based on the Dual Model of Grief, which postulates that normal grief is characterized by an ongoing fluctuation between restoration-oriented responses and loss-oriented responses. Being developed specifically for patients with advanced illness, this scale does not focus on somatic symptoms of depression, which generally overlap with expected symptoms of advanced illness and could generate false positives.

Palliative care clinicians must be aware that psychosocial variables and in particular cultural differences may decrease the likelihood that patients will admit to feeling depressed. For example, some patients with advanced illness may experience depression primarily as a somatic experience overlapping with symptoms of advanced illness and may have difficulty relating to the construct of depression as a psychological experience. Also, the presence of cultural stigma related to depression may prevent certain patients from feeling comfortable admitting they are feeling depressed. The concern that family members and treating physicians will feel disappointed if depression is present may prevent some patients from admitting to it. Additionally, language barriers may prevent patients from fully understanding what the construct "depression" refers to. In these and similar situations, palliative care and other providers will benefit from utilizing a clinical interview as a diagnostic tool, to supplement screening tools.

The palliative care team should carefully consider all available treatment options when caring for patients with advanced illness are suffering from depression. While prevalent in the palliative care setting, depression should not be considered a normal part of advanced illness. It should be actively treated, because it adds to the overall symptom burden and suffering experienced by patients and caregivers, at a time when the goals of the treating and palliative care team are to minimize distress and facilitate peaceful transitions and meaningful connections.

Antidepressant medications and psychostimulants may have an important role in treating depression in patients with advanced illness. Goals of treatment, side effect profile, drug interaction, and patient's prognosis are important considerations that guide clinicians in their choice of pharmacological agents. These issues have been reviewed elsewhere.[29]

It is important to remind readers that many palliative care patients who are very close to dying may become progressively less talkative, withdrawn, and disengaged. They may, in fact, appear depressed. They affect may appear flat, or they may appear pensive, yet not necessarily willing to discuss their emotions. This behavior may represent a change from a previous level of engagement and it may become a reason for concerns for family caregivers. However, in most cases this change represents yet another developmental stage for patients who are very close to death. As Kubler-Ross put it "Acceptance should not be mistaken for a happy stage. It is almost void of feelings". Thus, some terminally ill patients may begin a process of progressively withdrawing their emotional energy from external objects, situations, and even beloved family members. They may appear engaged in more internal, intrapsychic work, and less willing to engage. Yet, upon exploration, they generally deny feeling distressed. Unlike depression, this development is not pathological, and should be gently supported. Family caregivers who may feel hurt by the patient's disengagement will benefit from psycho education regarding the dying process. At this stage, it is important that they maintain emotional connection with the patient, while respecting his or her evolving needs.

Assessment of Complicated Grief

Research has shown that complicated grief, also called prolonged grief disorder (PGD), is a pathological response to bereavement associated with physical and psychiatric morbidity, including increased suicidal ideation and overall reduced quality of life (see Chapter 4 for a description). While a certain degree of symptom overlap exists, complicated grief is recognized as an entity different from PTSD and Major Depression.[33] The literature has focused discussion of complicated grief on bereaved individuals, where acute grief from the death of someone close is not integrated and causes severe and persistent pathology and disability.[33,34] However, it is important to remember that patients with advanced illness may also suffer from complicated grief for unprocessed losses that may have occurred several years prior.

Because of the suffering associated with complicated grief, identifying individuals at risk for developing complicated grief should be a particular focus of the palliative care team (Table 5.3). Factors described in the literature as exposing bereaved individuals to a higher risk for complicated grief include a childhood history of separation anxiety, overly controlling parent, parental abuse, early parental death, and insecure attachment styles. Additionally, a history of psychiatric illness prior to the loss and an ambivalent relationship with the deceased increase the risk for developing complicated grief and may seriously undermine patients and families' ability to cope with the progression of illness and impending death.[35,36]

It may be useful to group risk factors in categories related to (1) quality of the relationship and attachment style, (2) personal/familiar vulnerability, (3) circumstances of the death, and (4) psychosocial context of the death (see Table 5.5).

Table 5.5 Risk Factors for Complicated Grief

Relationship and Attachment style	Personal Vulnerability	Circumstances of the Death	Psychosocial Context of the Death
Anxious and ambivalent attachment High levels of dependence Childhood abuse and neglect	History of depression or other psychiatric illness History of unresolved losses Serious medical illness	Sudden, traumatic death Long, prolonged deaths	Lack of support during and after the death Financial stressors, including problems related to housing, insurance, access to care, etc.
Quality of relationship with the patient		• Previously estranged with recent attempt at reconciliation • Ambivalent • High levels of guilt for past events • Overly dependent and symbiotic	
Relationship with medical providers		• Antagonistic • Current lack of trust due to negative past experiences • Perception of abandonment by the medical provider • Fear of discrimination, racism, stigma	
Personal characteristics of the caregiver		• History of depression, anxiety, bipolar disorder, borderline personality disorder, substance dependence and abuse • Physical disability	
Circumstances of diagnosis/course of illness/death		• Patients diagnosed with advanced illness a few months before death • Sudden and unexpected death (e.g., sepsis neutropenia from chemotherapy) • Cause of death not directly related to illness patient is being treated for • Perception that illness/death could have been avoided	
Level of family/social support		• Social isolation • Dysfunctional family dynamics • Disenfranchised role	
Financial, related to health care system		• Inability to pay medical bills • Perception that financial difficulty is responsible for suboptimal care	

Table 5.6 Protective Factors for Complicated Grief
Emotional, practical preparation for the death of the patient
Adequate social support before and after the death
Supportive spiritual/religious beliefs

Identifying protective factors in patients and caregivers is equally important because these can mitigate the impact of risk factors (Table 5.6).

Complicated Grief In Clinical Practice

Symptoms of complicated grief include the following dimensions:[33,34,37,39]

- Separation distress, with intense longing and yearning for the deceased
- Anger and bitterness
- Shock and disbelief; Difficulty accepting that the loss has occurred
- Estrangement from others
- Hallucinations of the deceased
- Behavior change: Over involvement in activities related to the deceased, or excessive avoidance

In clinical practice, individuals with complicated grief may report disturbing dreams and intrusive images related to the deceased; preoccupation with the deceased and rumination about the circumstances of the death; they may be unable to recollect a full narrative of the circumstances of the death and may only be able to remember the most traumatic and disturbing images. Complicated grievers may utilize a significant amount of emotional energy to avoid thinking about the deceased, or to avoid places and situations that may be connected to the deceased. As individuals with complicated grief continue to experience disabling distress several years after the loss, they may no longer be able to identify the connection between their present distress and the loss. Thus, it is Important that clinicians always ask patients about previous losses and gently explore not only the meaning of the loss, but also how the grief has been integrated into the individual's psyche and current functioning. Individuals with complicated grief may initially present as depressed; however, research has shown that the dimensions mentioned above (yearning, anger and bitterness, shock and disbelief, estrangement from other, persistent hallucinations of the deceased, and behavior changes focused on avoiding or seeking connection with places and situations that remind of the deceased) represent symptom clusters unique to complicated grief.[42]

Complicated grief should be considered after the griever has been experiencing symptoms for over 6 month after the loss. However, the grieving process is unique to each individual. Some grievers have partially integrated acute grief six months after the loss; others will continue to the distress of normal grief for a longer period. However, while in normal grief the severity of distress gradually diminishes, in complicated grief clinicians may observe that grievers appear "stuck" in acute grief.

The Inventory of Complicated Grief (ICG), developed by Prigerson et al.[38] was developed to identify symptoms of complicated grief. It is widely used because of its psychometric properties supporting its validity and reliability and has been translated into several languages. Complicated grief is generally diagnosed when grievers score 30 or higher on the ICG at least six months after the death. As mentioned previously, complicated grief and major depression are different disorders, though they may be comorbid in the most severe cases.[39] Research has indicated that depression developed in the context of bereavement, also called bereavement-related depression, is not different from depression precipitated by other psychosocial stressors or endogenous factors.[40,41] Thus, it should be recognized and actively treated.

References

1. Hultman T, Reder EA, Dahlin CM. Improving psychological and psychiatric aspects of palliative care: the national consensus project and the national quality forum preferred practices for palliative and hospice care. *Omega (Westport)* 2008;57(4):323–39.

2. Screening and assessment. http://www.ncbi.nih.gov/bookshelf/br.fcgi?book=hssa mhsatip&part=tip51.ch4. Retrieved August 10, 2012.

3. Strada EA. The helping professional's guide to end of life care. Oakland, CA:New Harbinger, 2013.

4. Agnew A, Manktelow R, Taylor B, Jones L. Bereavement needs assessment in specialist palliative care: a review of the literature. *Palliat Med* 2010;24(1):46–59.

5. Ling SF, Chen ML, Li CY, et al. Trajectory and influencing factors of depressive symptoms in family caregivers before and after the death of terminally ill patients with cancer. *Onc Nurs Forum* 2013;1(4):E32–40.

6. Tang ST, Chang WC, Chen JS, et al. Course and predictors of depressive symptoms among family caregivers of terminally ill cancer patients until their death. *Psychooncology* 2012;27:3141.

7. Mosher CE, Bakas T, Champion VL Physical health, mental health, and life changes among family caregivers of patients with lung cancer. *Oncol Nurs Forum* 2013;40(1):53–61.

8. Northouse LL, Katapodi MC, Schafenacker AM, Weiss D. The impact of caregiving on the psychological well-being of family caregivers and cancer patients. *Semin Oncol Nurs* 2012;28(4):236–45.

9. Johansson AK, Grimby A. Anticipatory grief among close relatives of patients in hospice and palliative wards. *Am J Hosp Palliat Care* 2012;29(2):134–8.

10. Theut SK, Jordan L, Ross LA, Deutsch SI. Caregiver's anticipatory grief in dementia: a pilot study. *In J Aging Hum Dev* 1991;33(2):113–18.

11. Johansson AK, Sundh V, Wijk H, Grimby A. Anticipatory grief among close relatives of persons with dementia in comparison with close relatives of patients with cancer. *Am J Hosp Palliat Care* 2013;30(1):29–34.

12. Pomeroy EC, Garcia RB. The grief assessment and intervention workbook: a strength perspective. Belmont, CA: Brooks/Cole; 2009.

13. Cheng JO, Lo RS, Chan FM, Kwan BH, Woo J. An exploration of anticipatory grief in advanced cancer patients. *Psychooncology* 2010;19(7):693–700.

14. Cheng JO, Lo R, Chan F, Woo J. A pilot study on the effectiveness of anticipatory grief therapy for elderly facing the end of life. *J Palliat Care* 2010;26(4):261–9.

15. Marwit SJ, Meuser TM. Development and initial validation of an inventory to assess grief in caregivers of persons with Alzheimer's disease. *Gerontologist* 2002;42(6):751–65.

16. Mystakidou K, Tsilika E, Parpa E, Galanos A, Vlahos L. Screening for preparatory grief in advanced cancer patients. *Cancer Nurs* 2008;31(4):326–32.

17. Mystakidou K, Tsilika E, Parpa E, Katsouda E, Sakkas P, Soldatos C. Life before death: identifying preparatory grief through the development of a new measurement in advanced cancer patients (PGAC). *Support Care Cancer* 2005;13(10):834–41.

18. Mystakidou K, Tsilika E, Parpa E, et al. Illness-related hopelessness in advanced cancer: influence of anxiety, depression, and preparatory grief. *Arch Psychiatr Nurs* 2009;23(2):138–47.

19. Tsilika E, Mystakidou K, Parpa E, Galanos A, Sakkas P, Vlahos L. The influence of cancer impact on patients' preparatory grief. *Psychol Health* 2009;24(2):135–48.

20. Jacobsen JC, Zhang B, Block SD, Maciejewski PK, Prigerson HG. Distinguishing symptoms of grief and depression in a cohort of advanced cancer patients. *Death Studies* 2010;34(3):257–73.

21. Block SD. Assessing and managing depression in the terminally ill patient. ACP-ASIM End-of-Life Care Consensus Panel. American College of Physicians - American Society of Internal Medicine. *Ann Intern Med* 2000;132(3):209–18.

22. Bennett J, Berndt N, Hunter L. Issues in bereavement: preparatory grief vs. depression. *S D Med* 2008;Spec:41–42.

23. Chochinov HM, Wilson KG, Enns M, et al. Desire for death in the terminally ill. *Am J Psychiatry* 1995;152;1185–91.

24. Wilson KG, Chochinov HM, McPherson CJ, et al. desire for euthanasia or physician assistend suicide in palliative cancer care. *Health Psychol* 2007;26:314–23.

25. McCabe MP, Mellor D, Davison TE, Halford DJ, Goldhammer DL. Detecting and managing depressed patients: palliative care nurses' self efficacy and perceived barriers to care. *J Palliat Med* 2012;15(4):463–7.

26. Endicott J. Measurement of depression in patients with cancer. *Cancer* 1984;53;2243–8.

27. Little L, Dionne B, Eaton J. Nursing assessment of depression among palliative care cancer patients. *J Hosp Palliat Nurs* 2005;7(2):98–106.

28. Periyakoil VS, Hallenbeck J. Identifying and managing preparatory grief and depression at the end of life. *Am Fam Physician* 2002;65(5):883–90.

29. Widera EW, Block SD. Managing grief and depression at the end of life. *Am Fam Physician* 2012;86(3):259–64.

30. Holtom N, Barraclough J. The Hospital Anxiety and Depression Scale (HADS) useful in assessing depression in palliative care? *Palliat Medi* 2000;14:219–20.

31. Chochinov HM, Wilson KG, Enns M, et al. Are you depressed? *Am J Psychiatry*

32. Periyakoil VS, Kraemer HC, Noda A. et al. The development and initial validation of the terminally ill grief or depression scale (TIGDS). International Journal of Methods in Psychiatric Research. 2005;14(4):202–212.

33. Kacel E, Gao X, Prigerson H. Understanding bereavement: What every oncologist practitioner should know. *J Supp ort Oncol* 2011;9:172–80.

34. Zisook S, Shear K. Grief and bereavement: What psychiatrists need to know. *World Psychiatry* 2009;8(2):67–74.

35. Shear K, Shair H. Attachment, loss, and complicated grief. *Dev PSychobiol* 2005;47:253–67.

36. Silverman GK, Johnson JG, Prigerson HG. Preliminary explorations of the effects of prior trauma and loss on risk for psychiatric disorder in recently widowed people. *Isr J Psychiatry Relat Sci* 2001;38:202–15.

37. Simon NM, Wall MM, Keshaviah A, et al. Informing the symptom profile of complicated grief. *Depress Anx* 2011;28:118–26.

38. Prigerson HG, Maciejewski PK, Reynolds CF. Inventory of Complicated Grief: a scale to measure maladaptive symptoms of loss. *Psychiatry Res* 1995;59:65–79.

39. Sung SC, Dryman MT, Marks E, et al. Complicated grief among individuals with major depression: prevalence, comorbidity, and associated features. *J Affect Disord* 2011;134(1–3):453–8.

40. Kessing LV, Bukh JD, Bock C, et al. Does bereavement-related first episode depression differ from other kinds of depression? *Soc Psychiatry Psychiatr Epidemiol* 2010;45(8):801–8.

41. Kendler KS, Myers J, Zisook S. Does bereavement-related major depression differ from major depression associated with other stressful life events? *Am J Psychiatry* 2008;165(11):1449–55.

42. Ogrodniczuck J, Piper W, Joyce AS, et al. Differentiating symptoms of complicated grief and depression among psychiatric outpatients. *Can J Psychiatry* 2003;48(2):87–93.

Chapter 6

Psychosocial and Psychological Interventions for Grief Reactions

Focus Points

- Psychological interventions for grief reactions include supportive education, counseling, and grief-focused psychotherapy, each addressing varying degrees of symptom intensity and severity.
- Indication for treatment should be based on assessment of needs and existing risk factors, rather than on a general goal to prevent distress.
- Palliative care patients experiencing preparatory grief should receive adequate psychological support to process advanced illness and approaching death.
- All palliative care clinicians are encouraged to provide patients and families with psychoeducation and support and identify those who need specialized psychological and psychiatric intervention.

Patients' and caregivers' experience and expression of grief should be recognized, validated, and supported by palliative care providers and other health care professionals. Since grief and bereavement care is a mandated part of care, it is expected that each member of the interdisciplinary team will be involved, from the unique perspective of each discipline. Interdisciplinary care is particularly valuable because grief reactions and bereavement are shaped by multiple social, cultural, psychological, biological, and spiritual variables. While there is ample evidence that patients with advanced illness may experience high levels of preparatory grief, the grief and bereavement literature has primarily focused on studying grief interventions for bereaved individuals. In the last few years, studies have questioned the effectiveness and the benefit of bereavement support as a general preventive intervention offered to all grievers.[1-3] However, some have argued that the criticism of grief counseling was not based on sound evidence.[4] It is also possible that the methodological limitations of studies intending to show improvement may have affected outcome. In particular, very few studies of bereavement interventions clarify the theoretical bases and development of the interventions. Since the uniqueness of the grieving process has been established, it is not surprising that general interventions that do not specifically focus on the individual may not show dramatic results. For example, while participation in bereavement support groups is generally offered to grievers, it may not be the best match for the individual's style. Additionally, according to the Western psychological paradigm, counseling and psychotherapy generally rely on the verbal modality and emotional expression as vehicle for addressing distress and psychopathology. Clearly, these modalities may not resonate with members of other cultural groups or individuals whose grief processing is not based on the traditional model of "grief work," and may in fact be counterproductive. On the other hand, psychotherapeutic interventions targeting grievers with significant risk factors and grievers with high levels of distress have shown to be effective in improving symptoms.[5] However, while interventions developed for treatment of complicated grief were effective in reducing symptoms, preventive interventions did not yield significant results.[6]

Grief and bereavement research has highlighted several key points. (1) With enough social and family support, most bereaved individuals do not require professional help to integrate the loss and continue on with life. (2) Effective grieving does not necessarily require strong expression of emotions or distress, or prolonged "grief work." (3) Bereaved individuals who appear to be coping without expressing strong affect should not be forced to "talk about their feelings," but should be supported in a manner which is congruent with their own personal grieving style. (4) Patients and family caregivers experiencing anticipatory grief and bereavement can benefit from supportive grief education about grief reactions, including a discussion about the range of severity that can be expected. (5) Grief counseling should made be promptly available to patients and caregivers before the death of the patient, and to bereaved caregivers in the presence of significant risk factors, and in absence of adequate social, family, and community support. (6) Grief-focused psychotherapy and medication evaluation should be provided to individuals who develop pathological grief reactions, such as complicated grief (prolonged grief disorder) and bereavement-related depression, anxiety disorders, substance abuse, or other psychiatric disorders.

The Continuum of Interventions for Grief Reactions

It may be helpful to consider the range of available psychosocial and psychological interventions as distributed along a continuum of care. Clinicians should provide the appropriate level of care based on the several variables described in the assessment section (Chapter 5), including intensity and pattern of symptoms, availability of family and social support, and preexisting and current risk factors, without ignoring patients and family members personal preferences about treatment (Table 6.1).

Supportive Grief Education
Patient and family education about grief reactions is the first level of intervention. Many patients and caregivers are not aware of the symptom severity that is possible in normal grief and will benefit from communication with clinicians

Table 6.1 Psychological Interventions for Grief Reactions	
Supportive Education	• It can be provided anytime to patients and caregivers.
	• It explains the nature of normal grief and describes common symptoms that can be experienced.
	• It helps clarify and normalize patients' and caregivers' experiences.
	• It can help patients and caregivers recognize own individual grieving style and make sense of the constellation of symptoms experienced.
	• It may include referrals to primary care physicians and mental health professionals.
Counseling	• It is generally intended to facilitate normal grieving.
	• It may not benefit grievers whose symptoms would resolve on their own.
	• It generally includes psychoeducation.
	• Receiving it does not mean that pathology is involved.
	• It is generally focused on the "here and now" of the patient's experience and it generally does not address deep personality structures, trauma, or early childhood patterns.
Grief-focused psychotherapy	• It is a more structured intervention to address a complex grieving process, disenfranchised grief, or complicated grief (prolonged grief disorder).
	• It can explore the current grieving process in light of early childhood experience, trauma, complex relationships, and attachment patterns.
	• It may include referral to primary care physician for medication evaluation.

who validate and normalize their experience. Caregivers need to be reassured that what they are experiencing may be, for the most part, a natural expression of their grief and the stress of caregiving.

Patients with advanced illness may need gentle education about the process of preparatory grief and the distress that may be involved. They may experience significant preparatory grief with related distressing physical, cognitive, and emotional symptoms. Therefore, supportive grief education may become an important intervention to support patients as they process their own grief.

Supportive education can be provided by different members of the interdisciplinary palliative care team and other clinicians; it involves answering questions about grief reactions and explaining in a supportive and empathic manner basic information to patients and caregivers about what grief is, how it can affect them, what the possible symptoms are, and why it is not a disease or a pathological process, even if it feels intensely painful. Education can effectively address questions and clarify myths and questions about grief expressed by patients and caregivers, for example, "I should not feel so much pain; I should be stronger"; "I cannot focus, concentrate, and my memory is worse; am I losing my mind?"; "I feel nothing—What is happening to me?"; and "I have faith in God and I should not be feeling so sad." Supportive grief education can help normalize common experiences in grief reaction, such as physical and mental exhaustion, insomnia or hypersomnia, disturbing dreams, digestive problems, or physical manifestations of anxiety. Supportive grief education can address individual grieving styles, explaining how each person has a unique way of experiencing and expressing grief that should be recognized and supported. Patients and caregivers will benefit from being helped recognize their personal grieving style and associated phenomenology as a necessary manifestation of normal grief. They can also benefit form being encouraged to recognize and respect the expression of family members' grieving styles, especially when different from their own.[7,8]

While supportive education is a valuable initial intervention, in some cases it may not be sufficient and counseling or psychotherapy may become necessary. An initial thought, such as "I should not be feeling this way; I should be stronger" may at times develop into a deeper negative belief that affects the individual's self-esteem and coping ability in significant ways, such as "I am weak and inadequate. I cannot make it. And I am feeling this way because there is something wrong with me." Patients and caregivers who are experiencing high levels of ambivalence in their relationship may become overwhelmed by feelings of resentment and guilt and may also need counseling and psychotherapy to address deeper and older family dynamics. In these and similar cases the level of interventions needs to address deeper beliefs and emotions. For this reason, it is necessary to regularly monitor the development and evolution of grief reactions, to ensure the appropriate level of intervention is being provided.

Grief Counseling

Some clinicians do not differentiate between the terms *counseling* and *psychotherapy*, using the terms interchangeably. Others have argued in favor of a difference in depth and purpose between grief counseling and grief psychotherapy.[9] For the purposes of this manual, grief counseling and grief psychotherapy are considered as two different psychological interventions addressing different levels of depth and symptom complexity as described by Worden.[9] Counseling is considered a psychological intervention aimed at helping bereaved individuals process the distress involved in normal grief, guiding them through the various emotional states. For example, according to Worden's Task model, grief counseling is aimed at helping the bereaved accept the reality of the loss, work through the pain of grief, adjust to a world without the deceased, and establish an enduring connection with the deceased and continue on with life. Once again, it is important to emphasize that not all grievers need counseling or will benefit from it, and clinicians' recommendations should be based on an assessment of needs and discussion with the patient, rather than on a general desire to prevent distress Additionally, it is possible that, for some grievers, receiving practical help at home, especially in the case of parents with children who have lost a spouse, may be more beneficial than inviting them to "talk about it," especially when they do not feel the need to or they do not feel ready to. Obviously, practical help and grief counseling are not mutually exclusive interventions. The main point to remember is that interventions should match patients and families' level of distress, individual grieving style, and cultural values. While there is evidence that most grief reaction resolve without professional help, clinicians should not assume that this is true for all individuals. Presence of risk factors, especially lack of community and social support may negatively affect even resilient individuals and complicate the grieving process.

Grief-Focused Psychotherapy Approaches

Virtually every traditional psychotherapy model can be adapted and refocused primarily on grief. This sections briefly reviews application of different psychotherapy models to grief reactions. Psychotherapy is understood here as a structured psychological intervention with clear theoretical foundation to address deeper and older issues that may complicate the grieving process, as well as significant risk factors.[9] Psychotherapy should also be considered in the presence of complicated grief and bereavement-related depression.

In recent years psychotherapy approaches have been specifically developed to assist those who are experiencing significant difficulty processing their grief, especially complicated grief. Generally, the various models carefully combine elements from cognitive-behavioral, psychodynamic, insight-oriented, and existential approaches to target grief symptoms in an effort to increase effectiveness. The main approaches that have been empirically studied are briefly reviewed here.

Grief-focused psychodynamic psychotherapy focuses on the exploration of the relationship with the deceased, assisting bereaved grievers process negative affect associated with ambivalence and other interpersonal difficulties. Generally based on the concept of "grief work,"[8] it also examines the griever's defense mechanisms, facilitating the development of more adaptive defenses to support the grieving process. Therapy is intended as facilitating the expression of grief also by identifying any factors that may inhibit the griever's response. For example, strong negative emotions, such as anger, guilt, or shame may be perceived as unacceptable by the griever and may prevent expression of affect. Exploration of these difficult emotions and their underlying cause is understood an important factor in facilitating normal grief.[10]

Cognitive-behavioral therapy can be particularly helpful when grievers feel unable to reengage in regular life activities. The cognitive-behavioral model values a collaborative relationship with the therapist. It helps the patient develop a personal sense of control over distressing thoughts and cognitive distortions ("I should have been able to convince my husband to go to the doctor sooner; it is my fault he was diagnosed too late"), which promote and maintain distressing emotions (guilt, resentment, self-hate) and maladaptive behaviors. It can address unsupportive beliefs systems or unprocessed feelings of guilt, anger, or resentment and help the griever develop and follow a behavioral plan that includes valued activities, minimizing maladaptive coping behaviors, such as drug and alcohol abuse.[18,19] One distinctive feature of complicated grief is the griever's impaired ability to retrieve autobiographic memories.[11] It has been suggested that ability to modify retrieval of autobiographic memories may be one mechanism by which cognitive-behavioral therapy can improve complicated grief symptoms.[12]

Sleep disturbances are well recognized consequences in late-life spousal bereavement and in complicated grief and have the potential to create severe disruption in griever's life, often negatively impacting the ability to process grief.[13] Additionally, while complicated grief treatment has shown to be effective in improving symptoms of complicated grief, sleep disturbances persisted after treatment, indicating the need for adjunctive treatment.[14] Cognitive-behavioral interventions have been shown to be effective in improving insomnia, without the dangerous adverse effects of hypnotics.[15] These non-pharmacological interventions generally include sleep hygiene, cognitive restructuring, stimulus control, and sleep restriction.[13]

A recent review has concluded that, while general bereavement interventions based on the cognitive-behavioral model are effective immediately following the interventions, they do not yield statistically significant result at follow-up.[16] More studies are needed to identify not only the interventions with overall and long-term positive impact on bereavement, but especially the components of treatment that are effective. However, when compared with supportive counseling, cognitive-behavioral therapy was more effective in improving symptoms of complicated grief.[17] Loss of a partner or a child, less treatment motivation, early discontinuation, lower education level and higher symptom severity prior to beginning of treatment were factors associated with worse outcome.[18]

Group therapy is one of the traditional treatment modalities used in bereavement, generally with encouraging results, especially with improvement in perceived social support.[20,21–24,47] One study has indicated that patients' personality characteristics, such as quality of object relations and psychological mindedness may impacts their response to time-limited interpretative or supportive group therapy.[46] Clinicians should remember that not all grievers benefit from the group setting; therefore, personal treatment should always be discussed collaboratively and patients' preferences elicited.

Time-Limited Psychodynamic Therapy

Developed by Horowitz, this is an empirically validated, 12-session intervention for complicated grief.[25,26] According to Horowitz's model, expression of grief follows phases common in the stress response: outcry, denial, intrusions, working through, and completion. According to this model, complicated grief results from poorly integrated and contradictory emotions and cognitions associated with the deceased that affect grievers' self-concept and therefore sense of identity. One of the goals of therapy is to develop awareness and integration of unresolved feelings, thereby developing a new meaningful sense of self.

Family-Focused Grief Therapy

Developed by Kissane et al.,[27,28] family-focused grief treatment is a six- to eight-session family therapy intervention aimed at reducing emotional distress and dysfunctional communication patterns among family members, while facilitating appropriate expression of emotions. The intervention starts with assessment of families in the palliative care setting using the Family Relationship Index, a measure designed to recognize the predominant interpersonal style present in the family to identify those at bereavement risk. Based on their level of expressiveness, cohesiveness, and conflict, families are described as intermediate, sullen, or hostile. According to the model, screening families at their entry in palliative care allows identification of those at risk for decompensating during and after the death of the patient. Family therapy is then provided to families at risk during palliative and end-of-life care and continues during bereavement. A recent study of recorded therapy sessions with distressed families has suggested that delivery of certain components of family therapy in the palliative are setting may present challenges for therapists. In particular, exploration of family conflict, conceptualization of a comprehensive treatment plan, and utilization of family mottos occur with less frequency in the course of the treatment. However, results also showed that family therapist can apply the majority of interventions included in the model.[29]

Complicated Grief Treatment

Developed by Shear and colleagues[30,31] this intervention is based on the Dual-Model of Grief,[32] which postulates that grievers experience both loss-oriented response and restoration-oriented responses during mourning (see Chapter 2 for an explanation of the model). Thus, complicated grief treatment (CGT) focuses attention both on loss-related symptoms and positive life goals and future plans. In a randomized control study comparing 16 sessions of the CGT to 16 sessions of interpersonal therapy in 83 participants over 16–20 weeks, CGT was associated with a higher improvement of complicated grief symptoms and a faster response. The beginning of treatment includes an educational component, with information about normal and complicated grief and the Dual Model of Loss. Trauma-like symptoms were targeted by imaginal and in vivo exposure techniques used for posttraumatic stress disorder. Elaboration of negative memories and adaptive reconnection with the deceased was promoted by Gestalt techniques, involving imaginal conversations with the deceased. Grievers also receive assignments between sessions, such as keeping a grief monitoring diary.[33] A recent study has explored the role of hyperarousal of the sympathetic nervous system in treatment outcome of complicated grief therapy, by assessing catecholamines levels before and after treatment. Results showed that patients with the highest levels of epinephrine before treatment demonstrated the highest levels of complicated treatment post treatment. These results suggest that catecholamines levels may affect complicated grief therapy outcome.[34] Future studies should explore this aspect further.

Rosner et al.[35] described the development of a treatment manual for complicated grief disorder. The treatment (CG-CBT), designed to provide between 20 to 25 therapy sessions consists of three phases. The initial phase is focused on creating therapeutic alliance, providing psycho education, and teaching grounding exercises. The second phase involves exposing patients to the most difficult memories and thoughts about the death, challenging dysfunctional thoughts and replacing them with more accurate factual information about the events. This phase includes Gestalt techniques, such as imaginal conversation with the deceased. The third phase of treatment is focused on facilitating integration of grief and reflection about hopes and plans for the future. The authors studied the effects of this intervention on 50 inpatients suffering from complicated grief and an axis I disorder, comparing it with treatment as usual in the control group. They found the intervention was effective in improving complicated grief symptoms, but it did not significantly affect mental distress and depressive symtpoms.[36] The authors interpreted the results as an indication that the treatment was effective in selectively targeting grief symptoms, which could have relevant implications for clinical practice.

Internet, Multimedia, and Virtual Reality-Based Interventions

While few studies exist on interventions specifically developed for bereavement and complicated grief, there exist several non-clinical websites that have allowed many grievers to establish an online community of peer support, based on sharing and validating grief experiences, providing resources, and sharing hopes for the future.[42,43]

Studies on treatment for depression and anxiety indicates that clinical internet-based and multimedia interventions yield results that are similar to interventions provided by a clinician.[37] In a preliminary case report[38] the therapist worked individually with a patient suffering from complicated grief from a psychodynamic framework that included multimedia elements. The treatment included assisting the patient in selecting pictures of her deceased father representing the most meaningful moments. The pictures were posted as a slide show with soundtrack on a password protected website, accessed by the patient, family members and friends. The patient reported improvement of complicated grief symptoms.

In another pilot study, a virtual reality environment has been used to provide an 8-session treatment for complicated grief.[39] The virtual reality environment allowed the therapist to customize and personalize the experience for each participant.

A manualized Internet-based intervention has resulted in improvement of complicated grief symptoms that was maintained at 18 months follow-up.[40,41] The intervention consisted of expressive writing assignments provided to the patient by a therapist over the Internet. This treatment model may be also described as part of general tele health approach, where the clinician directs treatment and the computer becomes the medium through which treatment is provided. A psycho-educational self-help internet tool based on Martin and Doka concept of grieving styles (see Chapter 3) had a positive impact on helping participants normalize grief.[45] The tool consisted of 89 webpages, 28 videos, 22 video clips and 7 voice-over clips. Results showed significant improvement on all three outcome measures: attitudes towards grief, self-efficacy, and state anxiety. Additionally, results showed users were satisfied with the tool and would recommend it to others. Another brief internet-administered intervention based on written disclosure was effective in reducing feelings of emotional loneliness, while it did not alter grief or depressive symtpoms.[44]

While more research is needed to draw conclusions on the feasibility and efficacy of internet – based interventions and other novel modalities, this areas of research is promising, because it may represent an attractive alternative to individuals who would not seek treatment otherwise because of fear of stigma, or presence of health issues that make travel problematic. Internet-based interventions, if effective, be also be especially helpful to individuals living in rural areas who face challenges accessing competent and affordable care.

To summarize, clinicians in the palliative care setting who are wondering if they should refer grieving family members to bereavement services should consider the following:

- Bereaved family members with significant risk factors and high levels of distress, or who are already experiencing complicated grief should receive specialist assessment and treatment.
- Bereavement-related depression should be actively treated. Data show that antidepressants may improve symptoms of bereavement-related depression and help grievers tolerate the distress that may be involved in grief therapy (see Chapter 7).
- Bereaved family members with no risk factors and adequate psychosocial support may or may not benefit from bereavement interventions. Recent studies are recommending against psychological treatment in such cases, where grief symptoms are likely to improve on their own.[3] However, determination of needs must be based on careful assessment and regular follow-up. In many cases, oncologists, palliative care clinicians and primary care physicians are in the best position to continue to gently assess grievers' level of functioning. Thus, they are encouraged to integrate periodic bereavement assessment as part of their work with patients.
- Bereaved family members who do not experience strong affect and process grief through modalities other than emotional expression may not benefit from traditional bereavement support based on the concept of grief work. Furthermore, they may actually find that approach counterproductive. Therefore, the interventions should match the griever's personality and grieving style.

While bereavement research is a rapidly evolving area, the evidence relative to the effectiveness of psychological and psychosocial interventions is still mixed. Future research should focus on identifying therapeutic elements in each therapy approach to develop targeted interventions for grievers with different styles and clusters of risk factors.

References

1. Jordan JR, Neimeyer RA. Does grief counseling work? *Death Studies* 2003;27:763–86.

2. Schut H, Stroebe MS. Interventions to enhance adaptation to bereavement. *J Palliati Med* 2005;8(Suppl 1):S140–7.

3. Mancini AD, Griffin P, Bonanno GA. Recent trends in the treatment of prolonged grief. *Curr Opin Psychiatry* 2012;25(1):46–51.

4. Larson DG, Hoyt WT. What has become of grief counseling? An evaluation of the empirical foundations of the new pessimism. *Prof Psychol Res Practice* 2007;38(4):347–55.

5. Currier JM, Neimeyer RA, Berman JS. The effectiveness of psychotherapeutic interventions for bereaved persons: a comprehensive quantitative review. *Psychol Bull* 2008;134(5):648–61.

6. Wittouck C, Van Autreve S, de Jaegere E, et al. The prevention and treatment of complicated grief: a meta-analysis. *Clin Psychol Rev* 2011;31(1):69–78.

7. Raphael B. The anatomy of bereavement. New York, NY: Basic Books; 1985.

8. Lindemann E. Symtpomatology and management of acute grief. *Am J Psychiatry* 1944;101:141–8.

9. Worden JW. Grief counseling and grief therapy (4th Edition). New York: Springer. 2009.

10. Clark A. Working with grieving adults. *Adv Psychiatr Treat* 2004;10:164–70.

11. Maccallum F, Bryant RA. Impaired autobiographic memory in complicated grief. *Beh Res Ther* 2010;48(4):328–34.

12. Maccallum F, Bryant RA. Autobiographical memory following cognitive behavior therapy for complicated grief. *J Behav Ther Exp Psychiatry* 2011;42(1):26–31.

13. Monk TH, Germain A, Reynolds, CF. Sleep disturbances in bereavement. *Psychiatr Ann* 2008;38(10):671–5.

14. Germain A, Shear K, Monk TH, Houck PR, Reynolds CF, Frank E, Buysse DJ. Treating complicated grief: effects on sleep quality. *Behav Sleep Med* 2006;4(3):152–63.

15. Carter PA, Mikan SQ, Simpson C. A feasibility study of a two-session home-based cognitive behavioral therapy-insomnia intervention for bereaved family caregivers. *Palliat Support Care* 2009;7(2):197–206.

16. Currier JM, Holland JM, Neimeyer RA. Do CBT-based interventions alleviate distress following bereavement? A review of the current clinical evidence. *Int J Cog Ther* 2010;3:77–93.

17. Boelen PA, de Keijser J, van den Hout MA, van den Bout J. Treatment of complicated grief: a comparison between cognitive-behavioral therapy and supportive counseling. *J Consult Clin Psychol* 2007;75:277–84.

18. Boelen PA, de Keijser J, van den Hout MA, van den Bout J. Factors associated with outcome of cognitive behavioral therapy for complicated grief: a preliminary study. *Clin Psychol Psychother* 2011;18(4):284–91.

19. Kavanagh DJ. Towards a cognitive-behavioural intervention for adult grief reactions. *Br J Psychiatry* 1990;157:373–83.

20. Joyce AS, Ogrodniczuk JS, Piper WE, Sheptycki AR. Interpersonal predictors of outcome following short-term group therapy for complicated grief: a replication. *Clin Psychol Psychother* 2010;17(2):122–35.

21. Piper WE, Ogrodniczuk JS, Joyce AS, Weideman R, Rosie JS. Group composition and group therapy for complicated grief. *J Consult Clin Psychol* 2007;75(1):116–25.

22. Ogrodniczuk JS, Piper WE. The negative effect of alexithymia on the outcome of group therapy for complicated grief: what role might the therapist play? *Compr Psychiatry* 2005;46(3):206–13.

23. Kipnes DR, Piper WE, Joyce AS. Cohesion and outcome in short-term psychodynamic groups for complicated grief. *Intl J Group Psychother* 2002;52(4):483–509.

24. Ogrodniczuk JS, Piper WE. Social support as a predictor of response to group therapy for complicated grief. *Psychiatry* 2002;65(4):346–57.

25. Horowitz MJ. Stress response syndromes. New York: Jason Aronson, 1976.

26. Horowitz MJ, Krupnick J, Kaltreider N, et al. Initial response to parental death. *Arch Gen Psychiatry* 1981;38:316–23.

27. Kissane DW, McKenzie M, Bloch S, Moskowitz C, McKenzie DP, O'Neill I. Family-focused grief therapy: a randomized, controlled trial in palliative care and bereavement. *Am J Psychiatry* 2006;163(7):1208–18.

28. Zaider T, Kissane D. The assessment and management of family distress during palliative care. *Curr Opin Support Palliat Care* 2009;3(1):67–71.

29. Gaudio FD, Zaider TI, Brier M, Kissane M. Challenges in providing family-centered support to families in palliative care. *Palliat Med* 2012;26(8):1025–33.

30. Shear K, Frank E, Houck PR, Reynolds CF 3rd. Treatment of complicated grief: a randomized controlled trial. *JAMA* 2005;293(21):2601–8.

31. Shear MK. Complicated grief treatment: the theory, practice, and outcomes. *Bereave Care* 2010;29(3):10–14.

32. Stroebe MS, Schut H. The dual process model of coping with bereavement: Rationale and description. *Death Studies* 1999;23:197–224.

33. Loebach Wetherell, J. Complicated grief therapy as a new treatment approach. *Dialogues Clin Neurosci* 2012;14:159–66.

34. O'Connor MF, Shear MK, Fox R, Skritskaya N, Campbell B, Ghesquiere A, Glickman K. Catecholamine predictors of complicated grief treatment outcomes. *Int J Psychophysiol* 2012;(6):613–17.

35. Rosner R, Pfoh G, Kotoucova M. Treatment of complicated grief. *Eur J Psychotraumatol* 2011;2:7995.

36. Rosner R, Lumbeck G, Geissner E. Effectiveness of an inpatient group therapy for comorbid complicated grief disorder. *Psychother Res* 2011;21(2):210–18.

37. Amstadter AB, Broman-Fulks J, Zinzow H, Ruggiero KJ, Cercone J. Internet-based interventions for traumatic stress-related mental health problems: a review and suggestion for future research. *Clin Psychol Rev* 2009;29(5):410–20.

38. Nesci DA. Multimedia psychodynamic psychotherapy: a preliminary report. *J Psychiatr Pract* 2009;15(3):211–15.

39. Botella C, Osma J, Palacios AG, Guillen V, Banos R. Treatment of complicated grief using virtual reality: a case report. *Death Studies* 2008;32(7):674–92.

40. Wagner B, Maercker A. An internet-based cognitive-behavioral preentive intervention for complicated grief: a pilot study. *G Ital Med Lav Ergon* 2008;30(3 Suppl B):B47–53.

41. Wagner B, Knaevelsrud C, Maercker A. Post-traumatic growth and optimism as outcomes of an internet-based intervention for complicated grief. *Cogn Behav Ther* 2007;36(3):156–61.

42. Swartwood RM, Veatch PM, Kuhne J, Lee HK, Ji K. Surviving grief: An analysis of the exchange of hope in online grief communities. *Omega* 2011;63(2):161–81.

43. Walter T, Hourizi R, Moncour W, Pitsillides S. Does the internet change the way we die and mourn? Overview and analysis. *Omega* 2011;64(4):275–302.

44. Van der Houwen K, Schut H, van den Bout J, Stroebe M, Stroebe M. The efficacy of a brief internet-based self-help intervention for the bereaved. *Behav Res Ther* 2010;48(5):359–67.

45. Domnick S, Irvine AB, Beauchamp N, Seeley JR, et al. An Internet tool to normalize grief. *Omega* 2009;60(1):71–87.

46. Piper WE, McCallum M, Joyce A, Rosie JS, Ogrodniczuk JS. Patient personality and time-limited group psychotherapy for complicated grief. *Intl J Grp Psychotherapy* 2001;51(4):525–52.

47. Ogrodniczuk JS, Joyce AS, Piper WE. Changes in perceived social support after group therapy for complicated grief. *J Nerv Ment Dis* 2003;191:524–30.

Chapter 7

Psychopharmacology for Grief Reactions

Focus Points

- Major depression, anxiety disorders, and complicated grief can be serious complications of grief reactions that need to be recognized and treated.
- The presence of symptoms that reach a subclinical threshold requires careful clinical assessment and judgment to determine whether the use of medication is indicated.
- Available evidence provides some support for the use of antidepressants in bereavement-related depression, anxiety disorders, and complicated grief. A combination treatment of psychotherapy and antidepressant medication has resulted in highest levels of improvement.
- Concerns that use of psychotropic medication in the context of bereavement interferes with the normal process of mourning have not been supported by evidence.

While grief is not a disease, a certain degree of distress is to be expected as a normal reaction to bad news such as receiving a diagnosis of life-limiting illness, advanced illness, a poor prognosis, or learning of the death of someone close.[1–3] Most bereaved individuals, with enough support from family and friends, are ultimately able to manage intense grief, integrate it into their life experience, and even grow emotionally and spiritually from it. Similarly, specialist-level palliative care coordinated with other providers can provide adequate support to patients with advanced illness processing preparatory grief and approaching death. However, some patients and caregivers may need additional support, such as grief-focused psychotherapy and psychotropic medications, to manage the intensity of their grief symptoms.[4,5] And, even though grief is not a disease, it can become one, if the pain of loss cannot be managed. The fear of jumping too quickly to a medicalization of grief should not prevent providers from requesting an evaluation from mental health professionals and primary care physicians, when there is sufficient concern. The main point here is that grief is as unique as are people, and the need to receive professional help should not be perceived as a stigma by patients and providers.

In addition to accurate assessment, ongoing follow-up is needed to recognize the development of severe anxiety, major depression, or complicated grief. The importance of frequent reevaluation needs to be emphasized because patients' and caregivers' risk level may change rapidly, requiring a timely reconceptualization of the need for interventions.[6–10] In patients with advanced illness weakened by treatment and progression of illness major depression and preparatory grief may coexist, highlighting the need for additional support, including grief therapy and medication to relieve anxiety and depression symptoms. Older patients, with superimposed risk factors, may be particularly vulnerable. Patients and family members without adequate social and emotional support, as well as those with a history of substance abuse, depression and anxiety, or other psychiatric illness require a thorough risk assessment. Family members exhibiting a highly distressing level of anticipatory grief before the death of their loved one may also be at higher risk after the death. In addition, it is well recognized that traumatic events (i.e., sudden or prolonged deaths) are not uncommon precursors to the onset of major depression. Attempts should be made to monitor their effect during each assessment. Asking specific questions about sleep, appetite, social interactions, work performance, energy level, hopelessness, unexplained crying, and suicidal ideation can help discover this.

Perhaps as important as any specific inquiry is the personal availability that a clinician manifests during the follow-up contact. Establishing trust through evident caring will facilitate the discovery of difficulties processing grief and give the patient implicit permission to reveal his or her most personal sorrows and fears.

If severe grief symptoms are evident and especially if symptoms are progressive, early referral for a medication evaluation may be beneficial. Patients with advanced illness who exhibit severe preparatory grief reactions will benefit from specialist palliative care consultation. A recommendation for severely distressed family members to visit a primary care physician may also be of value and should be considered early. Primary care physicians may be in the best position to evaluate the physical and emotional toll of severe grief as well as the need for psychological intervention and/or medication. It must be emphasized that the medical decision to use psychotropic medication should generally be coordinated with a program for counseling, or psychotherapy. The integration of medication and psychotherapy is evidence based and should be recommended, when indicated.

Following are two examples of scenarios clinicians may encounter in the palliative care setting, which help illustrate important issues that should be taken into consideration during patient assessment.

Case Example

A 70-year-old man had experienced the loss of his wife 3 years ago. Two years ago he was diagnosed with prostate cancer, which is now metastatic. The patient was recently told of the worsening of his illness. He presents now with depressed mood, tearfulness, emotional withdrawal, and poor eye contact. He reports that he cannot sleep because sleeping is "too much like being dead." He often complains that he is alone dealing with the illness and that "It is just not fair." The patient has adult children who are supportive and visit regularly, but his ability to engage with them is very limited. When he looks at his children, he becomes tearful and asks, "Where is your Mom? She should be here with me." The patient often talks about his deceased wife, stating that her death "feels like yesterday; I expect her to walk in the room any moment." He refuses to eat and spends a significant amount of time every day crying and calling his wife's name out loud. He often states, "I am not worried about the cancer; I just need my wife back and I will be ok."

From this brief case description it appears that the patient's distress is primarily related to two main issues: bereavement and grief related to the progression of illness. A thorough clinical interview is warranted to determine whether the patient is suffering from bereavement-related major depression, preparatory grief, complicated grief and whether medication is needed. From the preliminary information it appears that the patient may be suffering from more than one complication of grief reactions. While his bereavement is not acute, as he lost his wife 3 years ago, his comments reveal that he perceives the death as having occurred in the very recent past. This reaction is not unusual, as his ability to continue processing the grief of his bereavement was probably first compromised by his diagnosis of prostate cancer only 1 year after her death. Furthermore, the grief associated with the new diagnosis of his advanced illness can be considered as an acute traumatic stressor that has reactivated the intensity of the grief of bereavement for his wife. The diagnosis of his own life-limiting illness has become superimposed on the bereavement process. In this circumstance, there is not only a rekindling of prior grief of bereavement but also risk for rekindling grief from other sources and even more distant losses, resulting in a dangerous spiral into more severe morbidity. This example highlights the importance of exploring all the levels of grief reaction experienced by patients. Clinicians working with patients with advanced illness may have the tendency to focus on a patient's future or imminent death as the main source of grief distress for the patient and the family. However, clinical experience shows that many patients who have experienced the loss of a loved one previously may attribute most of their distress to the experience of bereavement. Therefore, it is important to consider that patients with advanced illness may experience multiple layers of potentially interacting grief at the same time, including complicated grief.

Case Example

A 50-year-old woman recently diagnosed with metastatic breast cancer had demonstrated good coping skills and generally good adaptation to the diagnosis. She is single, never married, and lives with her 78-year-old mother, who has been widowed for 15 years. Mother and daughter go together to all medical appointments and, when asked, the patient reports that her mother is her main source of support. The initial psychosocial assessment revealed that the patient had, in her early thirties, been the primary caregiver for her father during a long illness. While she initially denied any psychiatric history, she stated that when she turned 40 years old she started feeling very sad "all the time" and could not get out of bed for several weeks. Her doctor told her she was depressed and prescribed antidepressants for her. She took the medication regularly, and when she started feeling better after a few months, she stopped it. After that episode she denies any feeling of depression. She has a few friends from childhood, but she regards none as close and she sees none regularly. She reports that during childhood and adolescence, her mother was always very concerned that spending time with friends would distract her from her school work and was afraid of "bad company." As a result, the patient grew up with the belief that her parents are the only people she could trust.

Two months after the beginning of cancer treatment the patient presented to the hospital for her scheduled chemotherapy, appearing distressed, anxious, and tearful. The nurse initially noticed this during her preliminary medical evaluation. Upon inquiry, the nurse discovered that the patient's mother had died suddenly at home from a heart attack three weeks prior. A distant relative who lives in another state has come to spend a week with the patient, but she is planning on returning to her home in the next couple of days. The patient is referred for psychological assessment.

The patient reports that she is crying continually at home and is unable to sleep or eat. She states, "This is so painful I feel I am going to die. I cannot catch my breath." She admits that even though she thinks about dying she will not try to kill herself "because I don't have the courage." She reports that while she is awake at night, she can hear her mother calling her and she calls out to answer. She feels upset because her mother does not answer back. This is associated with feelings of intense fear and panic.

Referred to a bereavement group, she refuses, stating that no one can understand her pain and how close she was to her mother. She is also concerned that people in the group will make fun of her and gossip about her. She states that "there is no point" in continuing to receive chemotherapy now that her mother has died. She states spirituality and religion are not important to her and declines the offer to meet with a spiritual care professional. She is, however, quite willing to engage with the nurse on a one to one basis. Therefore, she is offered individual meetings with a clinician who can provide psychosocial support focused on grief and bereavement. Though reluctantly, she accepts.

The patient is experiencing acute grief and is still in the early phases of bereavement. While, at this stage, her symptoms can be considered part of the normal grief experience, there are several areas of significant concern. First, it appears that this patient is not able to access sources of support that are typically utilized by bereaved individuals in their grieving process. This patient lives alone, does not have support of friends, family, or community, and is currently undergoing breast cancer treatment. The stress of her treatment and its side effects may impair her ability to process grief. She is not willing to reach out for bereavement support because over the years and due to her secluded life she has developed the belief that she cannot trust people outside her family. Additionally, and perhaps most important, she is experiencing persistent disrupted sleep, marked decreased in appetite, and severe anxiety. The severity of these symptoms warrants at least a visit to her primary care physician and medication evaluation, even if only three weeks have passed since the death of her mother. In the early phases of normal grief the acute onset of severe symptoms is not rare and is usually manageable with support. However, the presence of vegetative and psychological signs suggesting the development of bereavement – related depression warrants closer monitoring at least. If the patient meets criteria for major depression, this should be actively treated with psychotherapy, or a combination of psychotherapy and medication.

Second, it appears that the patient has had at least one major depressive episode and is currently not on medication. Individuals who have had a major depressive episode have a high risk of recurrence, especially in the presence of severe psychosocial stressors. Therefore, it may be more reasonable to refer the patient for a medication evaluation to consider whether treatment is indicated for a developing depressive episode. In addition, despite the acuteness of her symptoms, pharmacological intervention may become particularly important if she continues to experience intrusive thoughts and regular auditory hallucinations, and if her anxiety appears debilitating.

Use of Psychotropic Medication during Acute Grief

There is little research available on the use of psychopharmacology for grief reactions. Among the main reasons for this is that grief reactions, including complicated grief are not considered defined diagnostic entities. As mentioned previously, complicated grief was proposed for inclusion in the DSM-5, but it has not been recognized as a separate disorder. It has been argued that the lack of recognized diagnostic entity of complicated grief necessarily translates into less funding and therefore fewer studies.[15]

Psychotropic medication should never be utilized to suppress grief or reduce manageable but intense expression of affect in mourners. As mentioned in other chapters, significant distress in the form of intermittent uncontrollable crying, anxiety, profound sadness, difficulty sleeping, and even temporary perceptual disturbances is to be expected for variable periods of time. These symptoms do not necessarily need to be addressed with medication. However, even in acute grief, and in absence of a diagnosable mental health disorder, cognitive and physical manifestations of grief may become unmanageable for some grievers, especially when important protective factors, such as social support are not available. For example, sleep that is significantly and persistently disrupted and severe anxiety that prevents mourners from being able to sustain desirable function may need to be addressed with a judicious and short-term use of benzodiazepines or hypnotics.[11] However, the use of benzodiazepines in bereavement has long been a source of controversy. A randomized controlled study of 30 older men who had lost a spouse or a partner were randomized to either 2 mg of diazepam as needed for up to three times a day, or to similarly packaged placebo in the course of the first 6 months of bereavement for a period of six weeks.[12] Results did not show any evidence of positive or negative impact of benzodiazepine on bereavement. Of note, participants in the control group showed more improvement of sleep disturbances.

A survey of primary care physicians[13] indicated that many commonly prescribe benzodiazepines when a patient reports the death of a loved one. According to the study, these physicians do not consider their prescribing practices questionable. However, they acknowledge that in many cases, discontinuing benzodiazepine use was problematic. Data showed that 20% of long-term benzodiazepine users were initially prescribed the medication for acute bereavement grief, but never stopped. This practice of freely prescribing benzodiazepines for the symptomatic relief of grief has been called into question and serious concerns have been raised about the potential for dependency and the possibility that benzodiazepines may actually worsen bereavement manifestations, especially sleep disturbances.[14] Therefore, there is no evidence to support prescribing benzodiazepines *immediately* after a patient describes symptoms of anxiety or difficulty sleeping. And, considering the potential risks involved in benzodiazepine use, especially in older patients, there is not clinical reason for prescribing them as a general preventive strategy as soon as a patient communicates to a primary care physician that he or she is bereaved. These aspects are especially relevant for primary care physicians, often involved in the care of patients who may present with persistent somatic complaints and emotional distress as manifestations of grief reactions. Thus, the clinical interview should always explore the presence of psychosocial factors, such as bereavement, which may explain the current complaints. The patient's complaints should be accurately explored and understood, with the goal of identifying issues that may be addressed by psychoeducation, support and other behavioral interventions. In normal grief reactions, non-pharmacological interventions should be the first line of treatment.

For example, patients who are acutely grieving may experience a constant sense of fatigue and exhaustion; in an attempt to improve their energy level, they may significantly increase caffeine intake, which in turn can cause anxiety and disturbed sleep. Other patients may attempt to relieve anxiety by binging on large amounts of fatty foods and sweets, which may also interfere with their sleep cycle. Alcohol binges are associated with early morning awakenings and rapid heartbeat, which can also disrupt sleep and induce anxiety states. Many patients may respond well to relaxation exercises, imagery, and self-hypnosis to improve sleep and decrease anxiety in acute grief. However, many nonpharmacological interventions often require regular practice in order to be effective. Severe and disabling anxiety and persistent disrupted sleep may prevent some patients from being able to practice relaxation exercises. Providing the patient with a relaxation or self-hypnosis CD that they can simply listen to before sleep or when they are feeling particularly anxious can facilitate the practice. However, some patients may still need medication short term to decrease the level of arousal to a manageable degree allowing them to engage in and benefit from nonpharmacological interventions.

Pharmacotherapy for Bereavement-Related Depression

Early concerns that pharmacological treatment of depression in the context of grief would negatively impact the ability to effectively process grief are not substantiated. While sparse an typically conducted on small samples of participants, the current evidence suggests that antidepressants are safe and moderately effective in improving depressive symptoms in the context of bereavement-related major depression,[18,19] and in complicated grief, though improvement of specific grief symptoms has been typically of a lesser degree. These results, though preliminary and needing further study are important, because bereavement-related depression has serious negative consequence on health and overall function, especially in the older population.[22]

An early pilot study explored the effects of desipramine on 10 bereaved spouses. Results after 4 weeks of treatment showed that 7 participants reported significant improvement of depression, while a smaller group also reported improvement in grief symptoms.[16] Another study investigated the effect of nortriptyline in 13 bereaved older spouses suffering from bereavement-related depression. Treatment was started an average of 11.9 months after the loss, though the range was wide (2–25) and continued for a median treatment time of 6.4 weeks. Results showed the medication was effective in improving depression, but less effective in improving grief intensity.[17] Reynolds et al.[18] conducted a randomized double-blind controlled study exploring the effect of nortriptyline and interpersonal therapy on 80 participants suffering from bereavement-related depression for 16 weeks of treatment. Results showed that participants who received a combination of therapy and medication had the highest level of improvement and the lowest attrition rate. Additionally, participants who received nortriptyline alone also achieved remission. However, the study failed to show significant effects of treatment on grief intensity. This study enrolled participants who were 50 or older. Future studies could investigate similar treatments in different populations of bereaved individuals. The effect of bupropion sustained release was studied on a sample of 22 bereaved spouses whose loss had occurred 6 to 8 weeks prior and who met criteria for a major depressive episode.[19] Results showed that participants' depressive symptoms and grief intensity improved. Unlike the prior studies, decrease in grief intensity reached clinical significance, but to a lesser degree compared to depression.

Another study focused the investigation of antidepressants on activities of daily living, both motor and process activities, in 10 older persons who met criteria for major depression following the death of a spouse and obtained a low score (10) on the Assessment of Motor and Process Skills (AMPS), indicating difficulty in these areas.[20] Participants were randomized to either sertraline, or nortriptyline. Results showed that participants in both treatment conditions experienced a significant improvement of depressive symptoms and both motor and process activities of daily living. The suggestion that antidepressant medication may significantly improve bereavement-related depression in older bereaved spouses at risk for depression and disability has important implications for clinical practice.

A case study[21] explored the impact of sertraline on distressing dreams occurring in the context of bereavement. The authors contended that distressing dreams might not only be an expected manifestation of bereavement, but also of major depressive disorder. In the case of a 63-year-old woman who had lost her mother 5 months prior, distressing dreams of her mother getting angry at her started occurring with daily frequency, causing severe distress, generalized fatigues, and insomnia. After a psychiatric interview determined that she met criteria for a major depressive episode, a course of 25 mg. sertraline was initiated with complete remission of depressive symptoms and disappearance of the disturbing dreams.

Pharmacotherapy for Complicated Grief

There are few studies that have focused on the pharmacological treatment of complicated grief. While antidepressants have demonstrated some efficacy in relieving complicated grief symptoms, results have consistently shown that depressive symptoms tend to improve earlier in the course of treatment. Additionally, patients may present with both bereavement-related depression and complicated grief, thus challenging the ability to clearly differentiate between grief and depression symptoms.

In an early study 15 participants experiencing traumatic grief and depression, received a combination of therapy for traumatic grief and paroxetine.[23] Their results were compared with a different group of participants receiving nortiptyline for bereavement-related depression. Results showed that paroxetine was effective in relieving both symptoms of traumatic grief and depression and demonstrated effectiveness comparable to nortiptyline. The impact of escitalopram was investigated in a case series of 4 female participants presenting with complicated grief, defined as a score equal or higher than 25 on the Inventory of complicated grief. The treatment continued for 10 weeks and results showed significant improvement.[24] Escitalopram was also studied in the treatment of 30 bereaved adults after the death of a close family member.[25] After a 12-weeks course of treatment the majority of participants achieved significant improvement of depression, with 52% of participants achieving remission. Significant improvement was also noticed in levels of complicated grief. Although studied in a small sample, escitalopram demonstrated effectiveness in improving distress from uncomplicated grief, bereavement-related depression, and complicated grief.

Thus, the current evidence provides some support for the effectiveness of antidepressant for improvement of bereavement-related depression. There is also some indication that antidepressants may improve complicated grief, though improvement is typically slower and of a lesser degree. Clearly, more prospective studies are needed to understand the role of antidepressants in complicated grief. One area that has received very little attention is the impact of a combined treatment of psychotropic medication and psychotherapy on complicated grief. While an earlier study failed to demonstrate a significant impact of antidepressants and interpersonal therapy on levels of grief intensity,[18] a more recent study found that bereaved individuals suffering from complicated grief who were on a stable dose of antidepressants were more likely to complete a course of complicated grief therapy and were more likely to respond to treatment.[26] Complicated grief therapy involves being exposed to and processing painful memories associated to the death of the loved one. Therefore, it is possible that antidepressant medication may affect grievers' ability to tolerate intense negative affect that may be elicited by the treatment, hence enhancing compliance. However, this study was not prospective, as participants were already on a stable medication dose prior to enrolling in complicated grief treatment. Thus, controlled prospective studies are needed to allow drawing conclusions.

Discussing Medication Should Be a Therapeutic Intervention

Even when clinically indicated because of symptom severity, patients may be reluctant to accept psychotropic medication to assist them in managing disabling emotional distress from grief reactions. There may be several reasons for this response that should be elicited and explored in depth as part of the clinical interview. For example, they may feel overburdened by the amount of medication they are already taking or they may have concern about possible side effects. Patients with advanced illness may already feel that their life is regulated by the administering of medication, which may reinforce a sense of loss of control. Therefore, even adding one more medication may feel intolerable.

Some patients fear that taking medication will change them, or that it is an indication they are "grieving the wrong way" or that there is something wrong with them. For example, they may think that taking medication is an indication that they are not resilient or strong enough. Culturally based beliefs about using medication to address mood symptoms may also result in resistance or poor compliance. Family members may also express resistance toward psychotropic medication in the context of bereavement.

Patients who share these concerns may resist talking about their distress to mental health professionals who have been consulted to assist the primary team in assessment and diagnosis. This is especially likely to occur if the patient develops the impression that the clinician wants to "fix things with a pill". This behavior should not come necessarily as a surprise because talking about emotions is often more difficult for patients than discussing physical symptoms related to the illness. It is important to emphasize, however, that psychological assessments are often best undertaken by a clinician with an established relationship that conveys receptive attention and caring. When this occurs, the patient is less likely to feel pathologized and develop the impression that the team thinks grief and suffering can be treated with "a pill." Even if patients are experiencing complicated grief or depression, medication should not be the only treatment offered. Medication can have a more effective role in alleviating the patient's suffering in conjunction with psychotherapeutic treatment modalities that address grief and the overall existential and spiritual suffering common in patients with advanced illness.

If it is felt that medication would be necessary, it is important that providers reframe the meaning of drugs in a positive manner, thoroughly addressing individual concerns and fears.

Talking to patients about medication should be understood as an opportunity for a therapeutic intervention as well. The help needed to accept medications in a positive and welcoming manner may take considerable effort, time, and follow-up. It may be helpful to consider a stepwise approach to discussing medication with patients, especially around sensitive issues such as bereavement-related depression and complicated grief.

The first step is to unfold belief systems around medication and bring them to full awareness. For example, patients may fear that accepting medication to help manage their emotional distress is a sign that they are losing control. Some patients may feel so depressed about their prognosis that they may resist the idea of treating emotional distress in order to have a better quality of life. One patient with advanced ovarian cancer who had recently lost her spouse and was feeling very depressed responded to the consultation liaison psychiatrist who recommended an antidepressant: "Why should I take another medication that is not going to help with my cancer? Is it going to make my cancer stop spreading? How is feeling better emotionally going to help me? I don't see the point." Other patients may hold the belief that medication to treat anxiety and depression are "emotional crutches" that will make them dependent and take away their ability to "deal with things"; therefore, they may refuse to consider the use even short term. Patients with a history of substance dependence or abuse may feel particularly strongly about the need to "face" their emotional pain without "crutches." Unfolding and exploring these beliefs is important because not only may they affect the patient's perception of medication, but they may also significantly affect compliance, even when medication is accepted.

The second step is to gently explore what patients are already doing to improve their emotional distress, acknowledging and validating their efforts.

The third step is to reframe use of psychotropic medication as an additional ally, when its use is indicated, in the difficult journey through illness or bereavement.

Some patients and caregivers may respond to the use of metaphors. One of my patients with advanced cancer who was also grieving the death of her only daughter, which occurred 5 years prior, compared living with her grief to being on a very steep hike and carrying a backpack full of heavy stones. Considering medication became warranted in light of her severe difficulty sleeping and depression that was preventing her from engaging fully in psychotherapy. She subsequently compared our psychotherapeutic work together to something that helped her take out some of the stones but also helped her become symbolically "stronger" and develop her "survivor's muscles" so that she could continue carrying the load. We worked on reframing medication as another ally that could also help remove stones from the backpack, lighten her burden, allowing her "muscles" to get "stronger." Patients are often concerned that accepting medication means that they are not grieving the right way or that they are not strong enough. Some patients have commented that they find symptoms of acute grief, such as severe anxiety, difficulty sleeping, and presence of nightmares as embarrassing. They sometimes say, "I thought I was stronger than that."

Thus, normalizing the use of medication if needed to help the patient manage distress in acute grief or in complicated grief can be a very important intervention. Sometimes it is important to explain in very simple terms how medications function to restore "balance."

To summarize, use of antidepressants and the short-term and judicious use of benzodiazepine and hypnotics should be considered to assist grievers who are experiencing severe anxiety or sleep disorders in the acute phases of grief. Additionally, antidepressants should be considered to treat bereavement-related depression and complicated grief. Early concerns that use of medication will "block" the natural grieving process are not supported by evidence. In helping grievers manage acute grief, complicated grief, or bereavement-related depression, treatment should be integrative and include a combination of counseling or psychotherapy and, when needed, medication. The fear of "medicalizing" grief should never prevent clinicians from offering the patient all available and evidence-based treatment options. Certainly, medicalization of the natural grieving process is undesirable and would not represent sound clinical judgment. However, a priori ideas that patients should never receive psychotropic medication to relieve grief symptoms are also counterproductive and not reflective of current standards of care. Personal agendas in this respect should be replaced by careful, thorough, and on-going assessment and targeted treatment. Perhaps most important, discussions about the possible need for medication require clinical sophistication and deep understanding of the patient's worldview.

References

1. Stroebe W, Stroebe M. *Bereavment and Health: The Psychological and Physical Consequences of Partner Loss.* Cambridge, England: Cambridge University Press; 1987.

2. Barton D. The process of grief. In: Barton D., ed. *Dying and Death: A Clinical Guide for Caregivers.* Baltimore, MD: William & Wilkins; 1977.

3. Zisook S, Schuchter S. Mulvihill M. Alcohol, cigarettes, and medication during the first year widowhood. *Psychiatr Ann* 1990;20(6):318–26.

4. Maddison D, Raphael B. Normal bereavement as an illness requiring care: psychopharmacological approaches. In: Golberg I, Malitz S, Kutscher AH, eds. *Psychopharmacological Agents for the Terminally Ill and Bereaved.* New York: Columbia University Press; 1973.

5. Zisook S, Irwin SA, Shear MK. Understanding and managing bereavement in palliative care. In: Chochinov HM, Breitbart W, eds. *Handbook of Psychiatry in Palliative Medicine.* 2nd ed. New York: Oxford University Press; 2009, pp. 202–16.

6. Shear MK, Simon MD, Wall MM, et al. Complicated grief and related bereavement issues for DSM-5. *Depress Anxiety* 2011;28:103–17.

7. Simon NM, Wall MM, Keshaviah A, et al. Informing the symptoms profile of complicated grief. *Depress Anxiety* 2011;28:118–26.

8. Kendler KS, Myers J, Zisook S. Does bereavement-related depression differ from major depression associated with other life events? *Am J Psychiatry* 2008;165:1449–55.

9. Maj M. Depression, bereavement, and "understandable" intense sadness: should the DSM-IV approach be revised? *Am J Psychiatry* 2008;165(11):1373–5.

10. Kessing LV, Bukh JD, Bock C, et al. Does bereavement-related first episode depression differ from other kinds of first depressions? *Soc Psychiatry Psychiatr Epidemiol* 2010;45(8):801–8.

11. Woods JH, Winger G. Current benzodiazepine issues. *Psychopharmacology* 1995;118:107–15.

12. Warner J, Metcalfe C, King M. Evaluating the use of benzodiazepines following recent bereavement. *British Journal of Psychiatry* 2001;178:36–41.

13. Cook JM, Marshall R, Masci C. et al. Physicians' perspectives on prescribing benzodiazepines for older adults: a qualitative study. *J Gen Intern Med* 2007;22(3):303–7.

14. Cook JM, Biyanova T, Marshall R. Medicating grief with benzodiazepines: physician and patient perspectives. *Arch Intern Med* 2007;167:2006–7.

15. Bui E, Nadal-Vicens M, Simon NM. Pharmacological approaches to the treatment of complicated grief: rationale and a brief review of the literature. *Dialogues Clin Neurosci* 2012;14:149–57.

16. Jacobs SC, Nelson JC, Zisook S. Treating depression of bereavement with antidepressants. A pilot study. *Psychiatr Clin North Am* 1987;10(3):501–10.

17. Pasternak RE, Reynolds CF 3rd, Schlernitzauer M, et al. Acute open trial of nortriptyline therapy of bereavement-related depression in late life. *J Clin Psychiatry* 1991;52(7):307–10.

18. Reynolds CF 3rd, Miller MD, Pasternak RE, et al. Treatment of bereavement-related major depression in later life: a controlled study of acute and continuation treatment with nortriptyline and interpersonal psychotherapy. *Am J Psychiatry* 1999;156(2):202–8.

19. Zisook S, Schuchter SR, Pedrelli P, Sable J, Deaciuc SC. Bupropion sustained release for bereavement: results of an open trial. *J Clin Psychiatry* 2001;62(4):227–30.

20. Oakley F, Khin NA, Parks R, Bauer L, Sunderland T. Improvements in activities of daily living in elderly following treatment for post-bereavement depression. *Acta Psychiatr Scand* 2002;105(3):231–4.

21. Ishida M, Onishi H, Wada M, Wada T, Uchitomi Y, Nomura S. Bereavement dream? Successful antidepressant treatment for bereavement-related distressing dreams in patients with major depression. *Palliat Support Care* 2010;8(1):95–8.

22. Rozenzweig A, Prigerson H, Miller MD, Reynolds CF 3rd. Bereavement and late-life depression: grief and its complications in the elderly. *Annu Rev Med* 1997;48:421–8.

23. Zygmont M, Prigerson HG, Houck PR, et al. A post hoc comparison of paroxetine and nortriptyline for symptoms of traumatic grief. *J Clin Psychiatry* 1998;59:241–5.

24. Simon NM, Thomson EH, Pollack MH, Shear MK. Complicated grief: a case series using escitalopram. *Am J Psychiatry* 2007;164:1760–1.

25. Hensley PL, Slonimski CK, Uhlenhuth EH, Clayton PJ. Escitalopram: an open-label study of bereavement-related depression and grief. *J Affect Disord* 2009;113(1–2):142–9.

26. Simon NM, Shear MK, Fagiolini A, et al. Impact of concurrent naturalistic pharmacotherapy on psychotherapy of complicated grief. *Psychiatry Res* 2008;159(1–2):31–6.

Chapter 8

Grief-Related Distress in Palliative Care Teams

Focus Points

- Clinicians are not immune from experiencing grief in the course of their work with patients and are encouraged to find adaptive ways to express it and process it.
- Clinicians will benefit from recognizing the unique challenges and risk factors present in their work setting and develop protective factors accordingly.
- Professional self-care in the area of grief and bereavement includes developing an ongoing practice of self-awareness and recognizing one's own way of experiencing and integrating grief.

Palliative care involves accompanying patients and families during some of the most difficult times in their lives. Clinical work with patients and families during such a sensitive time requires the ability to create trusting relationships quickly, often by investing significant emotional energy into those relationships. This trust often creates a unique sense of belonging and closeness and, therefore, the development of attachment between patients and clinicians.

Thus, it should not be surprising that sharing such profound experiences may elicit sadness and grief in clinicians in the course of their relationship with their patients and after their patients' deaths. It is important that clinicians develop the ability to recognize and process their own grief in a manner that promotes integration and well-being. Otherwise, the inability to recognize and process feelings of sadness and grief when they occur may have a negative impact on clinicians' ability to connect meaningfully with patients. While palliative care professionals need to protect themselves from becoming emotionally overwhelmed by their patients' grief and distress, they should not become disconnected from their own grieving process. Grief is the normal reaction to loss; the nature of the palliative care setting may present clinicians with multiple opportunities to experience a sense of loss, and therefore a sense of grief.

Challenges and Risk Factors for Palliative Care Clinicians

Palliative care is now being provided in a variety of inpatient and outpatient settings (home, hospital, nursing homes), each presenting unique rewarding opportunities, but also challenges and risk factors.[1–4] It is important that clinicians reflect on the uniqueness of their professional work setting, be it a community hospital, a primary care physician's office, an outpatient clinic, or a hospice program.

For example, in the hospital setting, clinicians may find that a high number of inpatient consultations, while a positive indicator of service utilization, may also mean that there is very little time for emotional debriefing or other team-building activities. As a result, clinicians face the challenge of maintaining a sense of emotional balance as they move through such activities as discussing prognosis and goals of care, providing support to a dying patient or to the family of a patient who just died, sometimes without time for pause or reflection. Institutional demands may not allow enough time to acknowledge and process emotions individually or as a team. The emphasis placed on discharging patients not meeting acute care criteria may create pressure and conflict, at times undermining the trusting relationships carefully developed with patients and families. Discharge can be especially problematic on an emotional level if patients previously independent at home develop increased needs that warrant transfer to a nursing facility. Often these patients are admitted to the hospital to address acute needs, and then are no longer able to return to their homes. Their grief reaction can be intense and mirrored by that of clinicians who have been working very intensely to sustain their personal goals, as well as provide for their needs.[5–13]

Several clinical scenarios have the potential to elicit feelings of grief, frustration, disappointment, and even symptoms of anxiety and depression in clinicians. Reactions to challenging clinical scenarios are purely individual. Following are some examples that occur commonly:

• When financial, systems, insurance, and administrative issues create significant challenges for clinicians and it is felt that patient care is negatively affected as a result. While usually described in general terms as "systems issues", this aspect can have deleterious effects on team morale and productivity. For example, administrators may require that clinicians see a larger number of patients, which, in turns, requires spending less time with each patient. As a result, clinicians may feel that they are not able to able to provide the quality of care they desire. This may lead to professional dissatisfaction, sense of overwhelm, and burnout.

• When family meetings do not unfold as hoped and family members and/or patients express overt hostility and anger toward the team and/or each other, especially when it is felt that the team has somehow lost control of the meeting.

• When a significant amount of time and effort is given to a case and the outcome is perceived unsatisfactory.

• When several patients die within a short period of time (especially relevant in inpatient palliative care settings) and when the length of stay for patients in an inpatient unit is less than a day. This aspect can become especially relevant when a significant amount of time and energy has been allocated to facilitate a transfer to a palliative care unit from another institution or a different hospital floor and the patient dies either during transfer or a few hours after the transfer. In these cases, staff may have difficulty seeing the benefit of their efforts to facilitate the transfer and may experience a sense of futility.

- When the primary team does not follow recommendations of the palliative care team and it is felt that patient's suffering is increased as a result (e.g., it is felt that adequate pain management is not being achieved because of unwillingness to apply the recommendations of palliative care specialists).

- When the team experiences a "difficult death." This expression generally indicates situations where a patient's death has been marked by significant distress that has seriously affected all involved, including the clinical team. For example, this situation may occur when the relationship with the patient or the family has been particularly difficult, or particularly close, when it was felt that the patient was not managed adequately, or when the patient continued to experience significant suffering despite all efforts. A difficult relationship with a patient's family represents a well-known source of stress for the team.

Undeniably, the clinical setting presents clinicians with several opportunities for experiencing professional grief. The extent and the types of grief reactions depend on the particular work setting, clinicians' personality and history of past and present losses. Some clinicians may be more affected by the loss of the relationship resulting from the patient's death, while others may find the constant exposure to death and dying to be harder to manage. Other clinicians may have no significant difficulty with the emotional component of their work. However, they may feel very distressed by the administrative component of the work, especially when it affects patient care.[14–18]

It ensues that a first important step in professional self-care is developing awareness of stressors that can elicit grief reactions. However, heavy workload demands and the need to continue functioning effectively during the workday may prevent clinicians from acknowledging feelings of sadness, frustration, or grief. The suppression of emotions elicited during the work with patients may become an adaptive modality and often the main coping strategy during the workday. In palliative care, grief reactions related to work with patients often cannot be expressed due to situation and time constraints. Usually the decision to suppress is based on the perception "I shouldn't feel this bad" or "I just can't deal with this right now." Therefore, suppression can be a useful and sometimes necessary psychological defense mechanism to prevent distraction by the many thoughts and impulses that occur during the day. It permits focus and concentration on priorities. However, clinicians should find adaptive ways to recognize and process natural and expected emotional reactions, including grief reactions. Otherwise, these may become chronically suppressed and continue to accumulate.

Constant suppression and accumulation of grief and other emotions elicited by clinical work may become a significant risk factor, causing clinicians to avoid establishing emotional connections with patients, in an effort to protect their well-being. This approach would be especially problematic in palliative care, where patients and caregivers often need emotional support as much as they need pain and symptom management.

Accordingly, lack of awareness about what factors and situations have the potential to create distress is probably one of the most serious risk factors, because it prevents clinicians not only from recognizing negative impact of stressors, but also from developing the ability to do anything to ameliorate the situation. As obvious as this argument may sound, ignoring it may become surprisingly easy.

In the course of training clinicians develop expertise in helping patients when they are in distress. However, this does not necessarily mean they are also experts at recognizing and addressing their own emotional distress, when it occurs. Thus, self-awareness needs to be emphasized as a basic, but necessary skill for clinicians to recognize what emotions they are experiencing. Clinicians who cultivate self-awareness during the workday will be able to recognize when their physical and emotional energy level is off balance because of difficult emotions and states of mind. A moment of self-awareness and assessment can take only a few minutes and become an important tool for monitoring grief and distress throughout the day. A simple self-awareness strategy is to pause, take three deep breaths to quiet the mind, and acknowledge what one is experiencing in the moment. Recognizing and labeling feelings and emotions without judging them may become a simple, yet helpful strategy for clinicians to maintain emotional connection with themselves as well as patients and families. While clinicians may not be able to fully address their emotions and grief reactions during the course of the busy workday, awareness of their own needs may allow them to adequately address them at a more appropriate time. Suppressing strong emotions does not mean denying their existence; it means postponing processing the emotions at a later time, but acknowledging they are present.

Notably, whilst palliative care clinicians face various challenges, the literature suggests that, in general, working in palliative care may be a protective factor for burnout and psychiatric morbidity. For example, studies found that palliative care physicians report levels of psychiatric morbidity (depression, anxiety) similar to physicians in other specialties and less burnout.[19,20] Additionally, palliative care nurses reported levels of psychiatric morbidity similar to nurses working in other specialties, and lower levels of burnout. Compared to hospital nurses, hospice nurses reported lower levels of burnout.[21] However, the literature also indicates that palliative care professionals are not immune from experiencing psychiatric morbidity, which has a detrimental impact on their professional and personal well being.[22–26] Interestingly, a study exploring the presence of grief symptoms among long-term care staff found that the majority experienced at least one grief symptom. Staff who had been exposed to a greater number of deaths, despite having more professional experience, had more grief symptoms. And, the majority of staff reported they would have taken advantage of support for their grief reactions, if offered.[27]

Results from the literature notwithstanding, the experience of individual clinicians who may struggle to cope with the daily exposure to suffering, systems issues, and other challenges in the palliative care setting may not be fully captured by published studies. Therefore, as mentioned earlier, it is important that clinicians develop awareness of the unique challenges *they* may be facing personally, as well as their own personal risk factors.

The Interdisciplinary Team: Challenges and Opportunities

Mutual support provided by the clinical team members is extremely important in managing the stresses and challenges in palliative care work. During regular team meetings staff need to be provided with the opportunity to share difficult experiences and especially debrief difficult deaths. Discussing patients' deaths during team meetings should provide a meaningful opportunity to review some of the positive and negative aspects of working on each particular case. Responsibility to ensure this focus will depend on individual team members and importantly on skillful leadership. This is particularly necessary because poorly handled conflict among members, a persistent negative focus, and overall poor communication styles can create serious and ongoing distress in teams, making the daily life of its members particularly difficult.[28-30] Leadership needs to be attentive to mitigating the negative impact of conflict among team members as well as facilitating mutual support.[31-33] Implementing team-building activities that can promote a positive and supportive team culture should become a priority.

Managing Agendas and Expectations

While palliative care clinicians are committed to relieving patients' and care-givers' emotional and spiritual distress facilitating supportive family dynamics, they may inadvertently develop a preconceived concept of what represents a "good" dying experience. As a result, an agenda may be developed that includes goals not necessarily shared by the patients and the family, but idealized in the mind of the provider. For example, clinicians may wish to help patients and family members resolve old conflicts and reconcile prior to the death. However, the goals in these areas need to be identified by the patient. Clinical experience demonstrates that not infrequently, patients' goals may be far from forgiveness and reconciliation. Often, the palliative care setting offers only a snapshot in time of patients and families, which may hide a much more complex history. And, while it may not necessarily be conducive to reconciliations and expression of love and forgiveness in all cases, it may still allow for dignity and relative freedom from distress. Patients with advanced illness and approaching death benefit from experiencing a sense of physical and emotional safety. Identifying ways to promote a sense of safety in the midst of advanced illness and approaching death will allow clinicians to provide the level of integrative care that can benefit patients and families.[34]

Therefore, it is essential that clinicians first become aware of any personal agendas, hopes, or expectations in their work with patients. It is usually helpful and necessary to put them aside. Clinicians who are able to recognize and set aside their own preconceived notions and agendas will be able to welcome the patient and the family in an unbiased and non-idealized way, and authentically accompany them in the final portion of their unique journey.[35–37]

Countertransference

Palliative care clinicians develop close and empathic relationships with their patients. Working with particular patients may remind clinicians of past or current personal experiences with loved ones. As a result, clinicians may feel "pulled" to relate to patients in ways that, while understandable, may become counterproductive, because not based primarily on patients' needs, but on clinicians' unprocessed emotions. It is important that clinicians develop the ability to recognize, identify, and label their countertransference reactions. This will allow them to "step back" and reframe their relationship with patients in more therapeutic ways. Additionally, correctly identified and managed countertransference is not necessarily counterproductive and it can then be utilized to add depth to the clinical relationship.[38] Common countertransference reactions in the palliative care setting are as follows:

> The clinician may develop fantasies of symbolically "saving" the patient and may start making promises and raising expectations that are not realistic or appropriate. For example, a patient may wish to be discharged to a particular facility that cannot accept him or her because of insurance restrictions or the patient's medical needs. This type of situation is not uncommon in the palliative care hospital setting, and it certainly can evoke frustration in providers. However, the patient may become very distressed and ask the clinician to "save" him or her from the situation, by extending the hospital stay indefinitely, or convincing clinicians in charge of discharge planning that the plan is not acceptable. The clinician may start feeling as the only ally of the patient and the official "savior". This situation can create distress in the team and conflict between the palliative care team and the primary team, ultimately responsible for discharge planning.
>
> The clinician may start experiencing hopelessness or helplessness, sometimes mirroring the patient's own feelings of despair. There may be thoughts that nothing can be done to help the patient, and depression, death anxiety, and anticipatory grief may develop. As a result, the clinician may become ineffective. This type of countertransference may be elicited especially when working with patients who feel helpless and hopeless and patients who are experiencing severe depression. Additionally, clinicians who may have experienced a sense of hopelessness when caring for a family member with advanced illness may "project" similar emotions to a current clinical situation with a patient with similar circumstances.
>
> In other instances, the clinician may develop avoidance of the patient and the family due to the difficulty managing the intense emotional demands required by the situation. For example, the clinician may promise visiting and perhaps even offer a specific time just to pacify the patients and the

family, but he or she may then avoid the visit all together, eliciting feelings of frustration, abandonment, and anger in the patient and the family. This type of avoidance may also be the result of clinician's burnout, which can cause a sense of overwhelm in the professional.

As mentioned, particular patients may remind clinicians of their own family members and other loved ones with the same or similar medical diagnoses. Unprocessed grief for past losses on the part of clinicians may trigger powerful countertransference. As a result, they may start behaving "as if" patients were their own family members, thus compromising their ability to provide competent professional care.

Inability to recognize countertransference reactions as such have the potential negatively affect the working relationship with the patient and the family, as well as undermine personal and professional satisfaction. To deal successfully with countertransference reactions, there is first the need to recognize that a countertransference reaction is taking place; label the type of reaction experienced; and manage it, through awareness, clinical experience, and consultation with team members. Often, when the countertransference reaction is identified and acknowledged to another team member, it may immediately lose some of its emotional "power" on the clinician and allow for a more professional and reality-based approach.

Recognizing Burnout and Compassion Fatigue

Unprocessed and accumulated grief in clinicians may, with other factors, contribute to the development of burnout and compassion fatigue. Compassion fatigue, also known as vicarious or secondary traumatization, describes a condition developing when there is an imbalance between the amount of energy clinicians use to care for others and care for self.[39–44] A persistent lack of self-care when working in situations that constantly impose high emotional demands can create compassion fatigue, leaving clinicians feeling depleted and unable to continue connecting emotionally with their patients.

Burnout shares some aspects with compassion fatigue and reflects a condition of intense physical, emotional, and mental exhaustion from intense and persistent involvement in emotionally demanding situations. Burnout has the potential to create significant disruption in clinicians' professional lives. As a consequence, professional dissatisfaction can extend to clinicians' personal lives, threatening their entire sense of well-being.

Burnout can start as a slow and insidious process. It can be difficult to recognize, because in its early stages it often resembles a state of high activity, planning, and enthusiasm about professional and personal goals. This early stage is typically described as a honeymoon phase. In this phase clinicians may feel full of energy, with a strong desire to offer meaningful contributions to the work setting. However, ongoing stressful work demands may progressively undermine clinicians' ability to adequately cope. While compassion fatigue is primarily related to stress related to the clinical relationship with patients, burnout may be the result of external factors outside of clinician's control, such as longer work shifts that create difficult work conditions.[45–47]

The three main components of burnout are as follows:

- Emotional exhaustion
- Depersonalization
- Reduced sense of personal accomplishment

Emotional exhaustion can manifest as a sense of feeling drained, depleted, and without energy. Clinicians may become progressively irritable and angry, as well as feel depression and guilt for inability to establish and maintain emotional connection with patients, families, and other team members. The effort to continue functioning despite feeling emotional depleted may cause clinician to start resenting patients and family members for their needs and demands. As a result patients may be inappropriately and increasingly labeled as "difficult", when in fact the real difficulty is within the professional experiencing burn out.

Depersonalization involves objectifying patients, caregivers, team members and other clinicians, having lost the ability to connect with their humanity and vulnerability. The outward manifestation may include cynicism, feelings of resentment, and emotional withdrawal from patients and colleagues, as well as social withdrawal. Avoidance may develop at work. For example, in an institutional setting, clinicians may find they spend progressively less time visiting patients. They may become aware of their avoidance but rationalize it as caused by the busy schedule. In fact, burnout can make clinical work appear exhausting; as a result, clinicians may try to protect themselves from feelings of distress, by automatically decreasing their emotional involvement with patients. Other clinicians' work may be viewed cynically and constantly criticized. During team meetings, burnout may result in territoriality, difficulty collaborating with other team members, and numerous complaints about others, about the system, and about patients and caregivers, often without offering a solution or a sense of hope.

The third manifestation of burnout, reduced sense of personal accomplishment, or sense of being ineffective, may result in the development of a negative self-concept. Clinicians may develop feelings of decreased sense of worth and professional and personal inadequacy.

In essence, clinicians who are experiencing burnout may feel emotionally exhausted, "just tired of everything" and have lost a sense of connection to their work and their peers. The sense of emotional exhaustion may become combined with irritability, anger, avoidance, and a personal and professional sense of failure. Not surprisingly, burnout can become a risk factor for depression.

Self-Care Strategies

The importance of developing adequate self-care strategies to prevent grief overload, compassion fatigue and burnout cannot be overestimated. Clinicians should consider self-care not only as a professional and personal necessity, but also an ethical responsibility.[48–51]

Self-care should be considered an ongoing practice and should be developed to address clinicians' unique circumstances and stressors. Several studies and papers have described practices that have the potential not only to prevent distress, but also restore clinicians' professional and personal well-being once it becomes compromised.

The pleasure and sense of well-being that helping professionals experience when helping others has been called compassion satisfaction and it is considered a protective factor in burnout and compassion fatigue.[52] The ability to deeply and authentically connect emotionally with patients while maintaining adequate boundaries, has been named exquisite empathy.[53] It has been described as an important practice enhanced by the cultivation of self-awareness. Among ways to increase clinician's self-awareness are mindfulness meditation and reflective writing.[54] In particular, a study of 70 primary care physicians showed that intensive training in mindfulness meditation, communication, and self-awareness was associated with improvement in burnout and psychological distress.[55] Perhaps most importantly, clinicians will benefit from developing the ability to process professional grief and grief resulting from personal losses. Helpful strategies in this area range from peer consultation, supervision, and grief counseling, or psychotherapy. It is essential that clinicians recognize that, when grieving, they deserve the same level of attentive and compassionate care they strive to provide to their patients.

References

1. Fischberg D, Meier DE. Palliative care in hospitals. *Clin Geriatr Med* 2004;20:735–51.

2. Bennett M, Corcoran G. The impact on community palliative care services of a hospital palliative care team. *Palliat Med* 1994;8:237–44.

3. Morrison RS, Maroney-Galin C, Kralovec PD, Meier DE. The growth of palliative care programs in the United States. *J Palliat Med* 2005;8:1127–34.

4. O'Neil WM, O'Connor P, & Latimer EJ. Hospital palliative care services: three models in three countries. *J Pain Sympt Manag* 1992;7(7):406–13.

5. Becvar DS. The impact on the family therapist of a focus on death, dying, and bereavement. *J Marital Fam Therapy* 2003;29:469–77.

6. Berman R, Campbell M, Makin W, et al. Occupational stress in palliative medicine, medical oncology and clinical oncology specialist registrars. *Clinical Med* 2007;7(3):235–42.

7. Tilden VP, Thompson SA, Gajewski BJ, Bott MJ. End of life in nursing homes: the high cost of staff turnover. *Nursing Economics* 2012;30:163–6.

8. Peterson J, Johnson MA, Halvorsen B, et al. What is so stressful about caring for a dying patient? A qualitative study of nurses' experiences. *Intl J Palliat Nurs* 2010;16:181–7.

9. Larson DG. *The Helper's Journey: Working with People Facing Grief, Loss, and Life-Threatening Illness*. Champaign, IL: Research Press; 1993.

10. Worden W. *Grief Counseling and Grief Therapy: A Handbook for the Mental Health Practitioner* (3rd ed.). New York: Springer; 2002.

11. Rokach A. Caring for those who care for the dying: coping with the demands on palliative care workers. *Palliat Support Care* 2005;3:325–32.

12. Vachon ML. Staff stress in hospice/palliative care: a review. *Palliat Med* 1995;9(2):91–122.

13. Alexander DA, Ritchie E. Stressors and difficulties in dealing with the terminal patient. *J Palliat Care* 1990;6(3):28–33.

14. Grey-Toft PA, Anderson JG. Stress among hospital staff: its causes and effects. *Soc Sci Med* 1981;159:639–47.

15. Moon PJ. Untaming grief? For palliative care physicians. *Am J Hosp Pallliat Care* 2011;28(8):569–72.

16. Sansone RA, Sansone LA. Physician grief with patient death. *Innov Clin Neurosci* 2012;9(4):22–6.

17. Redinbaugh EM, Schuerger JM, Weiss LL, Brufsky A, Arnold R. Health care professionals' grief: a model based on occupational style and coping. *Psychooncology* 2001;10(3):187–98.

18. Papadatou D. A proposed model of health professionals' grieving process. *Omega J Death Dying* 2000;41(1):59–77.

19. Graham J, Ramirez AJ, Cull A, et al. Job stress and satisfaction among palliative physicians. *Palliat Med* 1996;10(3):185–94.

20. Dunwoodie DA, Auret K. Psychological morbidity and burnout in palliative care doctors in Western Australia. *Int Med J* 2007;37(10):693–8.

21. Masterson-Allen S, Mor V, Laliberte L, et al. Staff burnout in a hospice setting. *Hosp J* 1985;1:1–15.

22. Weinberg A, Creed A. Staff and psychiatric disorder in healthcare professionals and hospital staff. *Lancet* 1999;355:533–7.

23. Asai M, Morita T, Akechi K, et al. Burnout and psychiatric morbidity among physicians engaged in end-of-life care for cancer patients: a cross-sectional nationwide survey in Japan. *Psychooncology* 2007;16(5):421–8.

24. Taylor C, Graham J, Potts HWW, et al. The impact of hospital consultants' poor mental health on patient care. *Br J Psychiatry* 2007;190:268–9.

25. Payne N. Occupational stressors and coping as determinants of burnout in female hospice nurses. *J Adv Nurs* 2001;33(3):396–405.

26. Power KG, Sharp GR. A comparison of sources of nursing stress and job satisfaction among mental handicap and hospice nursing staff. *J Adv Nurs* 1988;13:726–32.

27. Rickerson EM, Somers C, Allen CM, Lewis B, Strumpf N, Casarett JD. How well are we caring for our caregivers? Prevalence of grief-related symptoms and need for bereavement support among long-term staff. *J Pain Symp Manage* 2005;30:227–33.

28. Parker GM. Cross-functional teams: working with allies, enemies, and other strangers. San Francisco: Jossey-Bass Publishers, 2003; pp. 37–97.

29. Hall P, Weaver L. Interdisciplinary education and teamwork: a long and winding road. *Med Educ* 2001;35:867–75.

30. Speck PW. Teamwork in palliative care: fulfilling or frustrating? New York: Oxford University Press; 2006.

31. Clark PG, Spence DL, Sheenan JL. A service/learning model for interdisciplinary teamwork in health and aging. *Gerontol Geriatr Educ* 1996;6(4):3–16.

32. Makaram S. Interprofessional cooperation. *Med Educ* 1995;29:65–9.

33. O'Brien PJ. Creating compassion and connection in the work place. *J System Therap* 2006;25:16–36.

34. Strada EA. The helping professional's guide to end of life care. Oakland, CA: New Harbinger Publications; 2013.

35. Brehony K. *After the Darkest Hour: How Suffering Begins the Journey to Wisdom*. New York: Owl Books; 2001.

36. Speck P. Working with dying people: on being good enough. In: Obholzer A, Roberts VZ, eds. *The Unconscious at Work: Individual and Organizational Stress in Human Service*. London: Routledge; 1994 Chapter 10, pp. 94–100.

37. Borrill C, West M, Shapiro D, et al. Team working and effectiveness in health care. *Brit J Health Care Manage* 2000;6(8):364–71.

38. Katz RS, Johnson TA. *When Professionals Weep: Emotional and Countertransference Responses in End of Life Care*. New York: Routledge; 2006.

39. Mackereth PA, While K, Cawthorn A, et al. Improving stressful working lives: complementary therapies, counseling and clinical supervision for staff. *Euro J Oncol Nursing* 2005;9:147–54

40. Fetter KL. We grieve too: one inpatient oncology unit's intervention for recognizing and combating compassion fatigue. *Clin J Onc Nurs* 2012;16(6):559–61.

41. Figley CR. Compassion fatigue: Psychotherapists' chronic lack of self-care. *J Clin Psychol* 2002;58:1433–41.

42. Pfifferling J, Gilley K. Overcoming compassion fatigue. *Family Pract Manage* Available at: http://www.aafp.org/fpm/20000400/39over.html. Accessed October 20, 2002.

43. Wright B. Compassion fatigue: how to avoid it. *Palliat Med* 2004;18:4–5.

44. Keidel GC. Burnout and compassion fatigue among hospice caregivers. *Am J Hospice Palliat Care* 2002;19:200–5.

45. Maslach C, Jackson SE. Maslach burnout inventory manual. 2nd ed. Palo Alto, CA: Consulting Psychologist Press; 1986.

46. Sherman DW. Nurses' stress and burnout. *Am J Nurs* 2004;104:48–56.

47. Stimpfel AW, Sloane DM, Aiken LH. The longer the shifts for hospital nurses, the higher the levels of burnout and patient dissatisfaction. *Health Aff* 2012;31(11):2501–9.

48. Mason C. Basic themes. In: Mason C, ed. *Journeys into Palliative Care: Roots and Reflections*. London: Jessica Kingsley; 2002, Chapter 1, pp. 15–30.

49. Jones SH. (2005). A self-care plan for hospice workers. *Am J Hospice and Palliat Med* 2005;22:125–8.

50. Pope, KS, Vasquez MJT. *Ethics in Psychotherapy and Counseling: a Practical Guide* (4th edition). Hoboken, NJ:Wiley; 2011.

51. Breiddal, SMF. Self-care in palliative care: A way of being. *Illness, Crisis, and Loss* 2012;20(1):5–17.

52. Stamm BH. Measuring compassion satisfaction as well as fatigue: developmental history of the compassion satisfaction and fatigue test. In: Figley CF (ed.) *Treating Compassion Fatigue*. New York, NY: Brunne-Routledge; 2002:107–19.

53. Harrison RL, Westwood MJ. Preventing vicarious traumatization of mental health therapists: identifying protective practices. *Psychotherapy* 2009;46(2):203–19.

54. Grossman P, Niemann L. Schmidt S, Walach H. Mindfulness-based stress reduction and health benefits: a meta-analysis. *J Psychosom Res* 2004;57(1):35–43.

55. Krasner MS, Epstein RM, Beckman H, et al. Association of an educational program in mindful communication with burnout, empathy, and attitudes among primary care physicians. *JAMA* 2009;302(12):1284–93.

Index

Page numbers followed by *t* indicate a table